Recent Advances in Bone Tumours and Osteoarthritis

Edited by Hiran Amarasekera

Published in London, United Kingdom

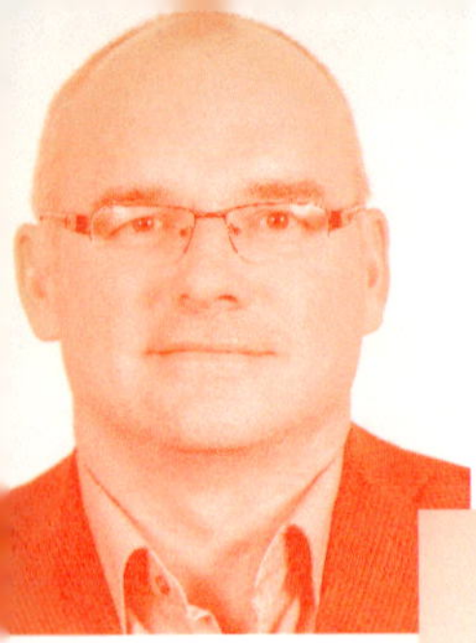
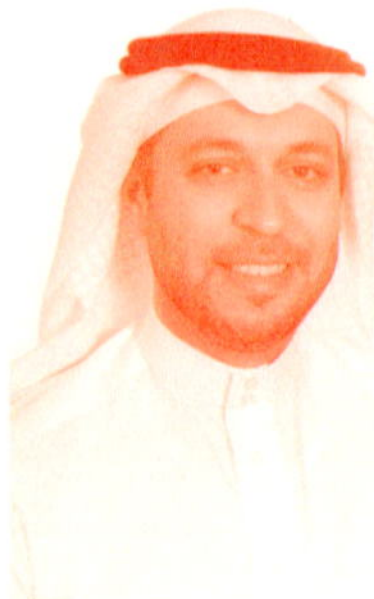
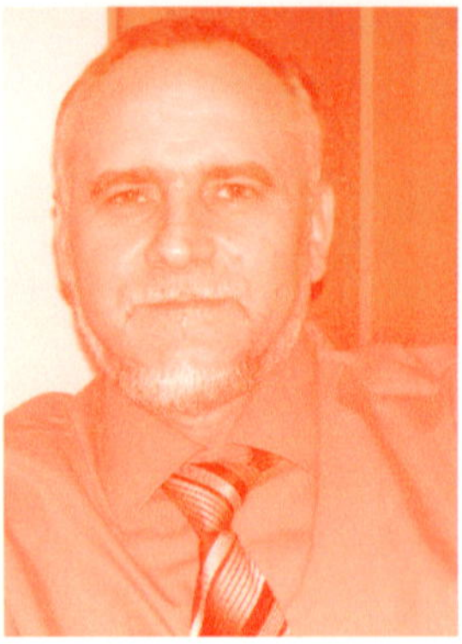
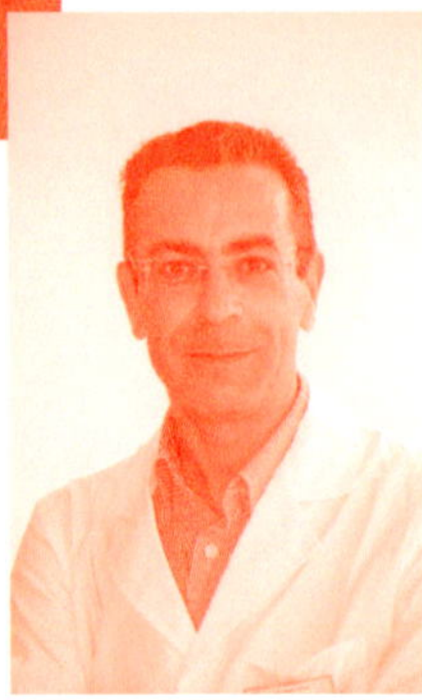
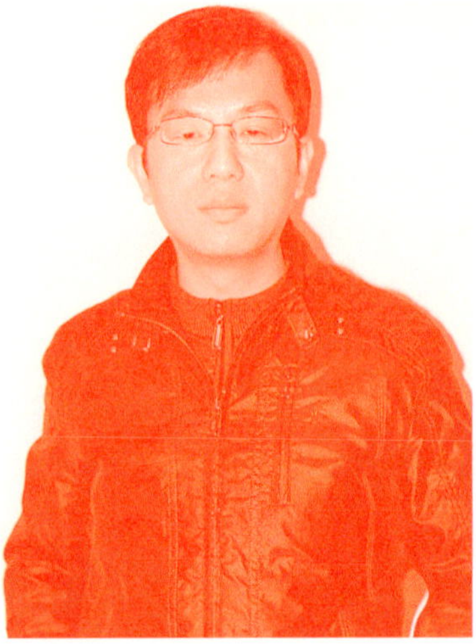
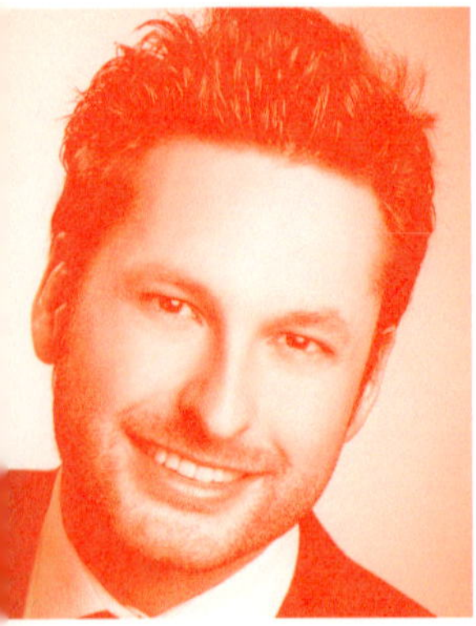
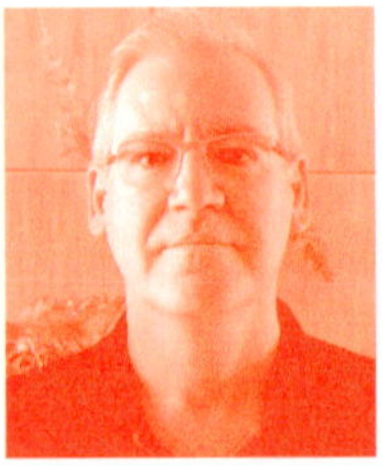

IntechOpen

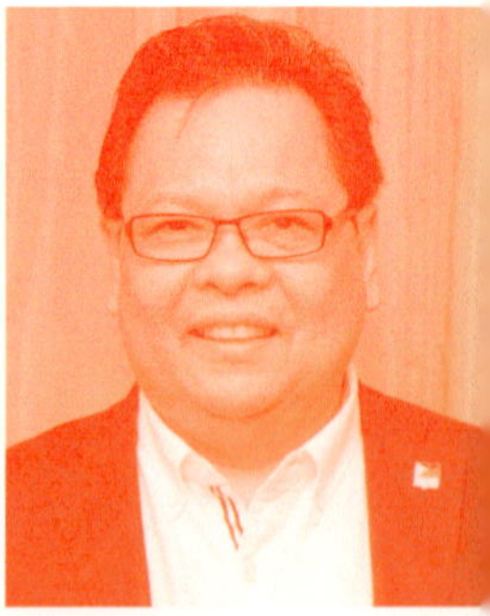
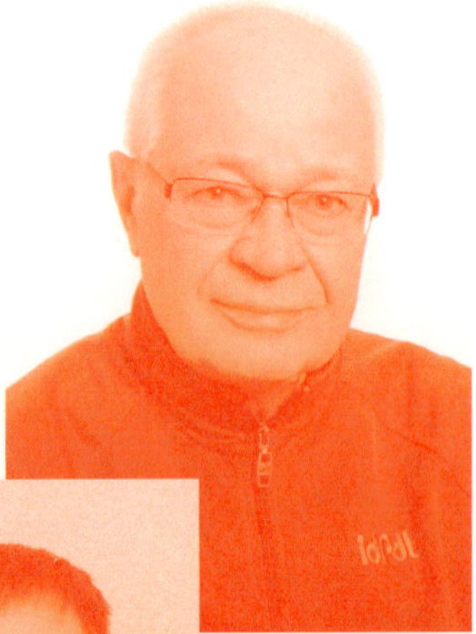
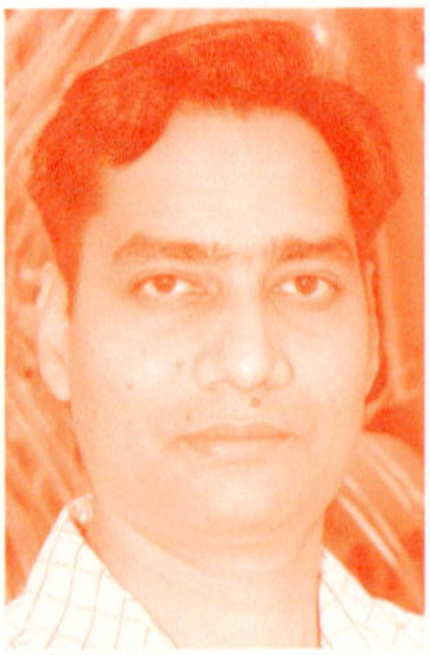
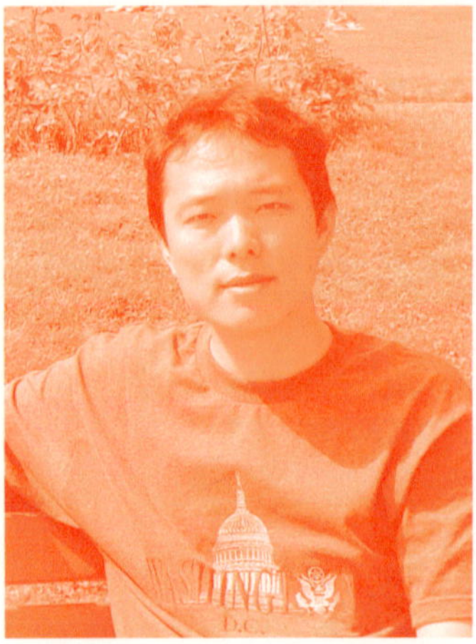
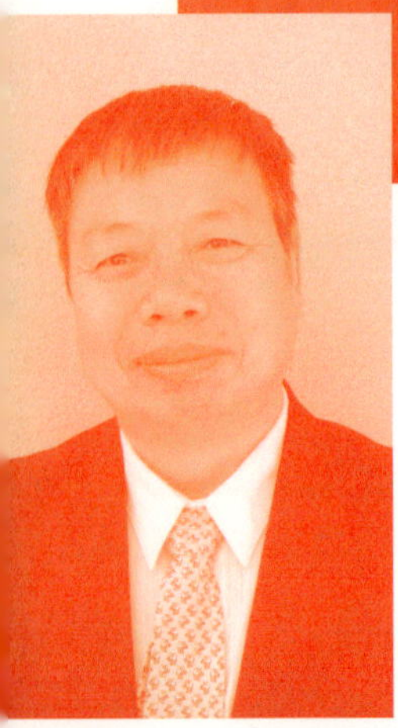
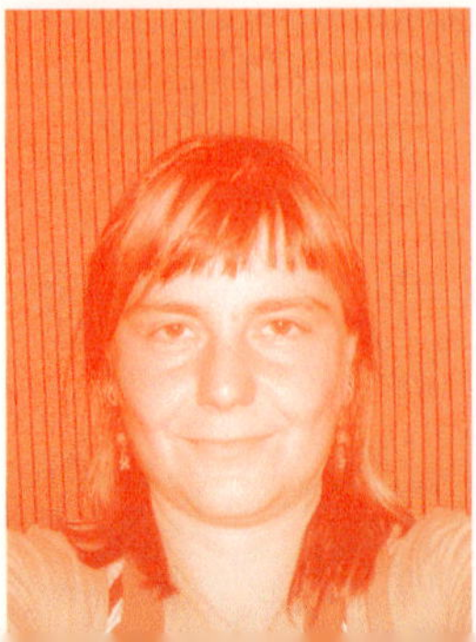

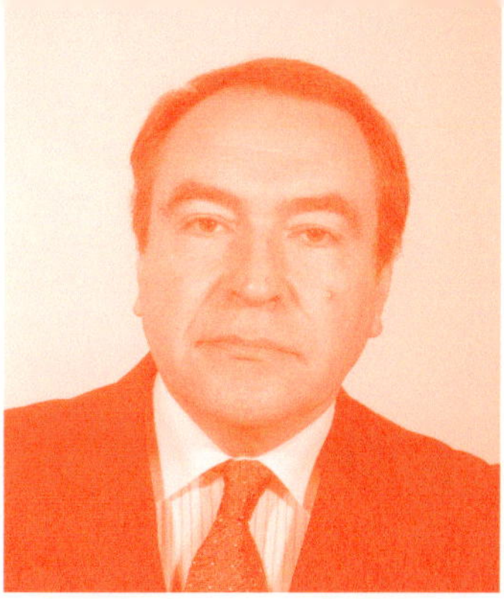
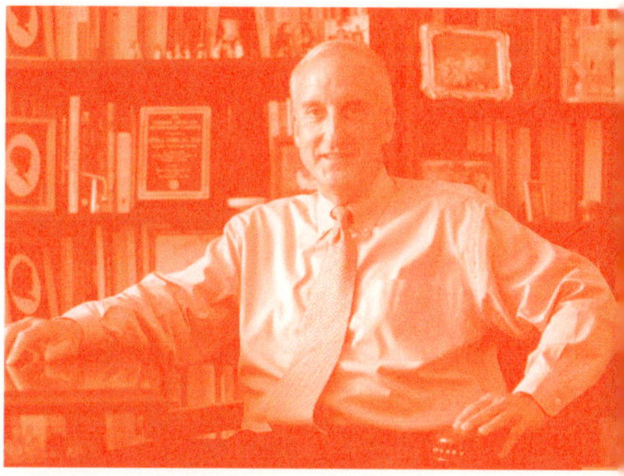
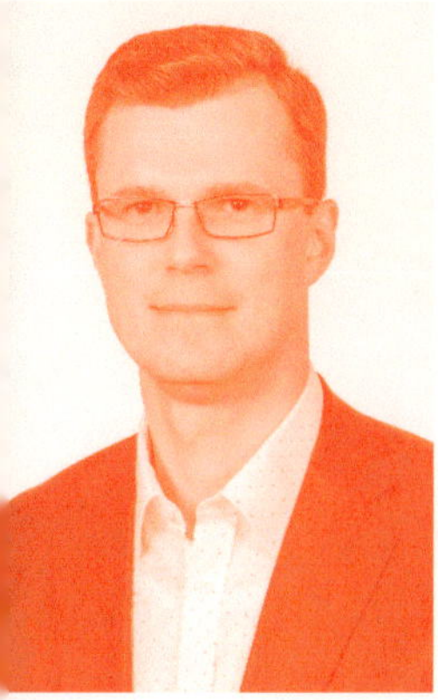
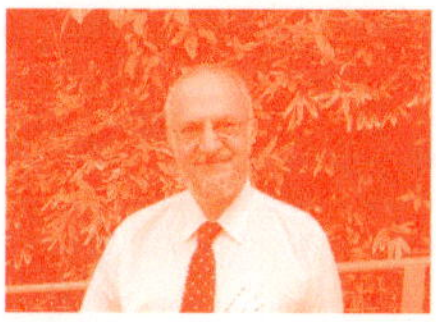
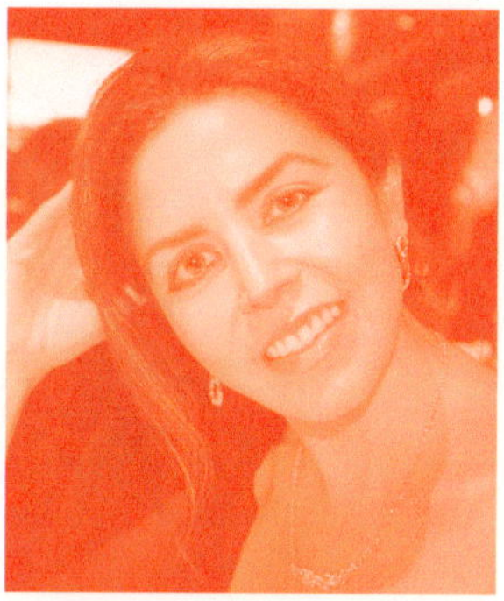

Supporting open minds since 2005

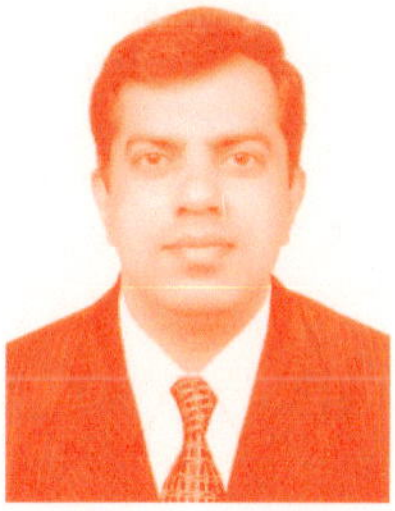
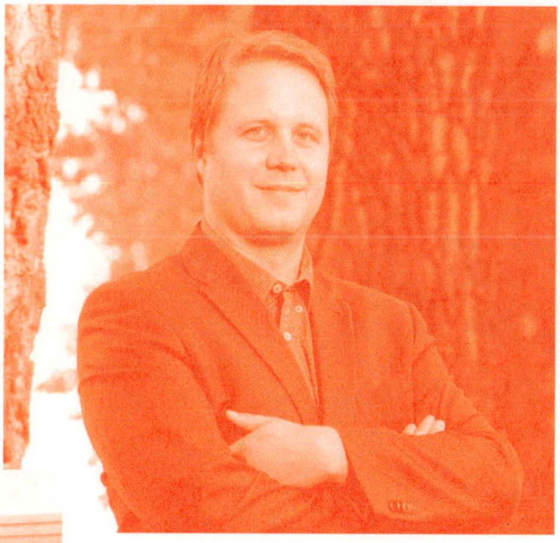
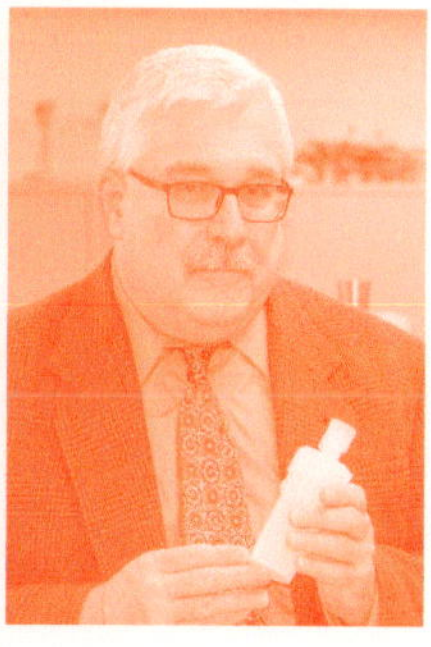
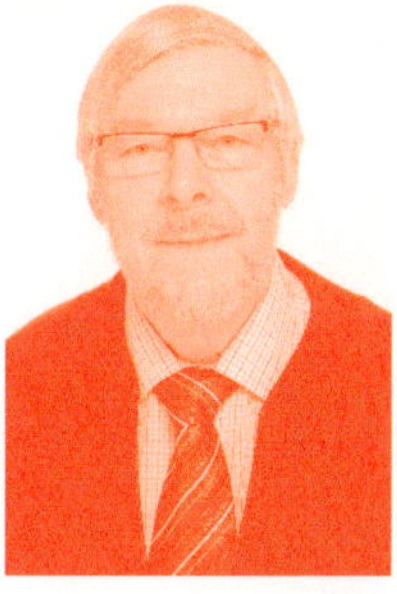
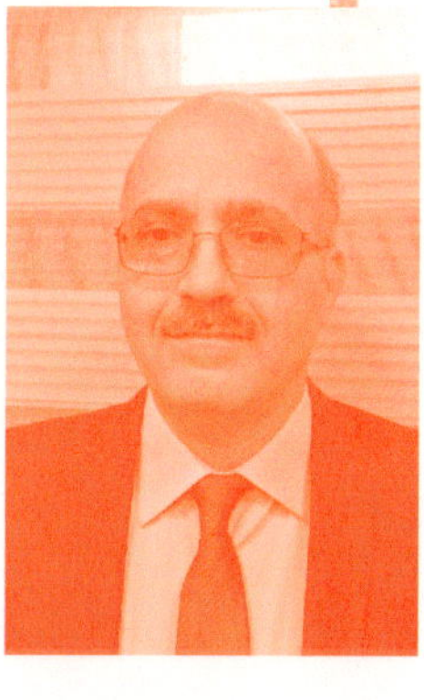
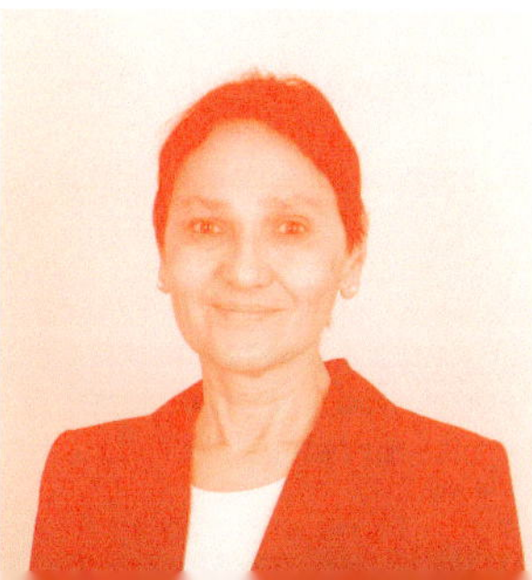
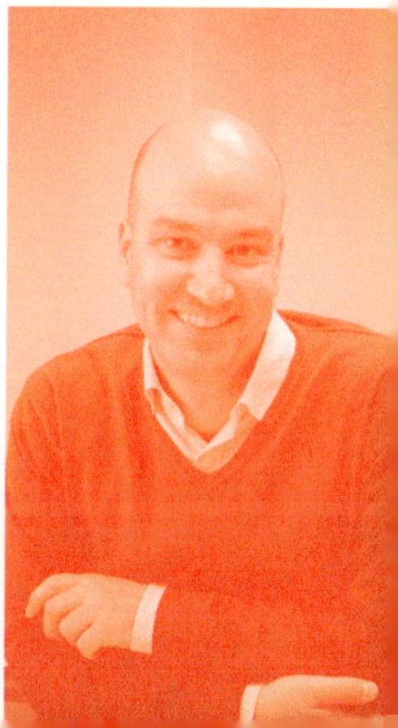

Recent Advances in Bone Tumours and Osteoarthritis
http://dx.doi.org/10.5772/intechopen.87284
Edited by Hiran Amarasekera

Contributors
Ahmed Mostafa Kotb Aziz, Charles Mackworth-Young, Harold Wilson-Morkeh, Aleksandar Radunovic, Ognjen Radunovic, Maja Vulovic, Milan Aksic, Aleksandar Matic, Recep Öztürk, Sonny Hermanus Johannes Hermanus Johannes Sliepen, Ana C. Belzarena, Gottardo Bianchi, Leticia Gaiero, Nicolas Casales, Claudio Silveri, Luis Costa, Isabel Fernandes, Raquel Lopes-Brás, Sandra Casimiro, Jignesh Shah, Ankita Chauhan

First published in London, United Kingdom, 2021 by IntechOpen
IntechOpen is the global imprint of INTECHOPEN LIMITED, registered in England and Wales, registration number: 11086078, 5 Princes Gate Court, London, SW7 2QJ, United Kingdom
Printed in Croatia

British Library Cataloguing-in-Publication Data
A catalogue record for this book is available from the British Library

Additional hard and PDF copies can be obtained from orders@intechopen.com

Recent Advances in Bone Tumours and Osteoarthritis
Edited by Hiran Amarasekera
p. cm.
Print ISBN 978-1-83968-923-9
Online ISBN 978-1-83968-924-6
eBook (PDF) ISBN 978-1-83968-925-3

For EU product safety concerns:
IN TECH d.o.o., Prolaz Marije Krucifikse Kozulić 3, 51000 Rijeka, Croatia, info@intechopen.com or visit our website at intechopen.com.

Meet the editor

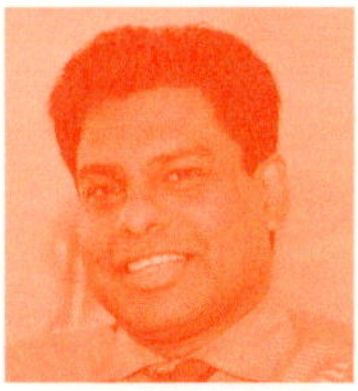

Hiran Amarasekera is a Consultant Orthopaedic Surgeon Currently practicing in Sri Lanka. After obtaining the MBBS from Kasturba medical college, Manipal, Inda, he completed the MS in Surgical sciences from the University of Colombo. He obtained the fellowship of the Royal College of Surgeons of Edinburgh (FRCS Ed) and board certification in 2003. His special interests are in the areas of young adult hip and knee problems, sports injuries, lower limb arthroplasty, and keyhole joint surgery, and revision arthroplasty. His present research is focused on non-surgical and minimally invasive alternative treatment for osteoarthritis. He worked and trained in many countries for over twenty including India, Sri Lanka, Australia, United States, and the UK. As a keen researcher, he has completed an MPhil from the University of Warwick and completed a research fellowship at the University of California Los Angeles, (UCLA). Presently, he works as a medical educator, as an honorary senior lecturer at the University of Kelaniya and Kothalawela Defense University in Sri Lanka. He is an examiner of medical students both in Sri Lanka and the UK and a course provider for Trauma courses run by the college of surgeons and was elected a fellow of Sri Lanka College of surgeons in 2013. Dr. Amarasekera is the editor of the Journal of Sri Lanka Orthopaedic association and council member. He is a reviewer for the Journal of Bone and Joint Surgery (Br) e and Bone and Joint Journal (BJJ) and a member of the editorial board of the Sri Lanka Journal of Surgery (SLJS). He has over 50 international publications, presentations and several book chapters to his credit and has reviewed over 100 papers for journals of BJJ and SLJS. After joining IntechOpen in 2012 he authored three book chapters and edited several open access books with them.

Contents

Preface

Management of bone tumors and osteoarthritis has evolved rapidly over the past years. The diagnostic capabilities, treatment modalities, treatment preferences, timing of treatment, and approach to managing these conditions have changed over the years.

This book contains two main sections. The first section contains chapters on recent advances in bone tumours and the second section contains chapters on the latest findings in osteoarthritis and its treatment.

Chapters are organised in a systematic way so the reader can review and understand the basic to advanced concepts of the subject. All chapters are original work contributed by an expert panel of authors and the work is peer-reviewed and edited accordingly.

The first section contains 5 chapters dedicated to bone tumours that discuss the recent advances and current management in bone cancer pain, imaging of paediatric benign bone tumours, medical therapy for giant cell tumours, osteosarcoma and its modern management.

The second section is dedicated to osteoarthritis where the authors discuss the timely topics of initial management, modern non-surgical treatment options and the role of bilateral joint replacements in a single sitting when treating osteoarthritis.

The book in printed format will be an essential reference to store in all medical libraries, while the electronic format in the open-access concept is available free of charge for the reader to read online or download, either the book in whole or as an individual chapter.

Sincere and many thanks to all the authors' contributors and researchers who contributed to this book and made this project a success, all the staff at Intech Open publishing including the author service manager, Jasna Bozic, for the effort put into this project, and as always to my wife Anuji and daughter Nuwanji, for supporting me through all my research work and helping with high tech computer editing.

Hiran Amarasekera
MBBS(Manipal), MS (Colombo), FRCS(Ed), FCSSL, MPhil (Warwick),
Consultant Orthopaedic Surgeon,
Senior Lecturer (Hon) In Surgical Sciences,
Faculty of Medicine,
University of Kelaniya,
Sri Lanka

Section 1

Bone Tumours

Chapter 1

Bone Cancer Pain, Mechanism and Treatment

Sonny Hermanus Johannes Sliepen

Abstract

The world health organization (WHO) has predicted a global amount of 19 million cancer cases by 2025. Breast, prostate and lung cancer are common cancer types and show metastasis in 60 to 84% of the cases, with 75 to 90% experiencing life-altering cancer-induced bone pain (CIBP), characterized by continuous, dull progressive pain with movement-induced incident peaks and random breakthrough spikes. Therefore, it is the most difficult pain condition to treat. CIBP is a unique type of pain with neuropathic and nociceptive components. Briefly, an invading tumor cell disturbs the healthy balance of the bone resulting in an acidic microenvironment, activating sensory fibers in the bone. The invaded tumor cell and adjacent stromal cells secrete mediators initiating an immune response with transcriptional signaling, resulting in increased cytokines and growth factors. Sensory nerve fibers are damaged and start to sprout, causing ectopic firing, and as tumors grow in size they activate mechanoreceptors. Aside from bisphosphonates and antibody therapy, CIBP is treated by a range of NSAIDs to strong opioids, but remains undertreated in one-third of cases. This chapter discusses the accompanying CIBP of bone tumors, the mechanism of action and current treatments.

Keywords: CIBP, NOP receptor, RANK/RANKL, NGF/TrkA, IL-6

1. Introduction

Cancer induced bone pain (CIBP) is a big accompanying clinical problem of bone tumors with a high unmet medical need [1]. It is a debilitating form of different pain components that severely affects a patients' quality of life. The complex mechanism of CIBP largely involves the nervous system with transmembrane receptors and channels on the nerve fibers. Briefly, the nervous system consists of the central nervous system, i.e. the brain and the spinal cord, and the peripheral nervous system, i.e. the autonomic (unconscious, the para- and sympathetic nervous system) and somatic (conscious/voluntary) nervous system. A neuron is a nerve cell consisting of a cell body (soma), projections receiving input signals (the dendrites) and a single long arm away from the soma (the axon/fiber) that ends with the axon terminal (synapse). Axons contain a sheath of myelin that serves as isolation in a similar way as plastic around an electrical wire. Regarding the somatic nervous system, neurons with projections towards the spinal cord (afferent) respond to stimuli and are the sensory neurons. The neurons that respond to the brain and the signals from the spinal cord (efferent) are the motor neurons [2].

Pain is the defense mechanism against external factors that could cause tissue damage (a noxious stimuli) and nociception is detecting such stimulus. The somatosensory nervous system contains the sensory neurons that respond to noxious stimuli (nociceptors). There are three types of nociceptors, receptors that sense 1) thermal, 2) mechanical and 3) chemical stimulants. When a threshold of either one of those three properties is exceeded, the nociceptor is activated – *the neuron depolarizes and an action potential occurs* – and an electrical signal follows through the nociceptive pathway. Two major nociceptive fibers are reasonably fast-conducting A-δ fibers, containing a thin layer of myelin and the unmyelinated slow-conducting C-fibers. Finally, there are thickly myelinated fast conducting A-β fibers, faster than A-δ fibers, primarily for the normal sensation of touch [2].

Pain can be acute, serving a biological purpose, e.g. protection, and chronic, without a biological purpose, becoming an own medical disease more than a symptom [3]. A workgroup from the international association for the study of pain (IASP) has defined chronic pain as a pain that persists for more than 3 months. They defined a subgroup in 2018 where it has been considered that pain can be the primary disease, i.e. in low-back pain. Moreover, they have made subgroups and considered conditions with chronic secondary pain, such as chronic cancer-related pain [4]. The transition to chronic pain involves neuronal plasticity – *the ability of the nervous system to adapt the composition, signaling and structure* – represented by the enhancement of neurons and pain pathways, entitled as central and peripheral sensitization [3]. A very detailed elaboration on the molecular mechanism of sensitization is described by Latremoliere and Woolf (2009). Here, it is important to know that central and peripheral sensitization is a mechanistic explanation for mechanical allodynia (*non-noxious stimuli become painful*), hyperalgesia (*painful, noxious stimuli are prolonged in response and exaggerated*) and secondary hyperalgesia (*pain spreads beyond the site of injury*) [3]. The definition of pain by IASP is: "*An unpleasant sensory and emotional experience associated with actual or potential tissue damage, or described in terms of such damage*" and for nociception: "*The neural processes of encoding noxious stimuli*" [5]. Pain can be distinguished between injury to the peripheral tissue, nociceptive pain – *Immunologic response* – and pain directly to the nervous system, neuropathic pain. IASP has defined neuropathic pain as: "*Pain caused by a lesion or disease of the somatosensory nervous system*". No specific definition is mentioned for nociceptive pain, however, chronic inflammation is a particular pain-related event, recognized by chemical and inflammatory mediators, affecting nociceptive axons and resulting in lowered thresholds of neuronal excitation [6]. CIBP is a unique type of pain with nociceptive and neuropathic components but the exact mechanism remains unclear.

This chapter elaborates on the mechanism of action of bone cancer pain. Next, a brief subsection of the bone anatomy & physiology. Finally, treatment options used for CIBP and bone metastases are described, including CIBP models to assess novel compounds and the mechanism of action.

2. Bone cancer pain

2.1 Bone anatomy, physiology and innervation

Bones can be classified by their shapes, i.e. flat, short, long and irregular bones [7]. The most common bones that encounter metastasis of tumor cells are long bones [8, 9], i.e. the tibia, femur and humerus, characterized by an extended tubular diaphysis and round-shaped distal and proximal epiphyses [10]. The outer part is covered with a fibrous layer and an inner osteogenic layer, the periosteum and cambium layer, respectively [11]. The latter contains progenitor cells for the bone building cells, osteoblasts [11]. Briefly, mesenchymal-derived cells are the progenitors which are stimulated by the transcription factors core binding factor α1 (Cbfa1), Osterix (Osx) and activating transcription factor 4 (ATF4) to initiate osteoblastogenesis [12]. Matured osteoblasts secrete bone matrix until they become resting osteoblastic cells (bone-lining cells) [7, 12, 13]. Behind the periosteum are densely packed tube-like structures called osteons (Haversian system). One osteon consists of several layers (lamella) with small gaps (lacunae) in between, containing nutrient transportation cells, osteocytes, constituting 90 to 95% of the bone cells present in the mature human skeleton [7, 13]. Osteocytes originate from differentiated bone-linings cells after they are encapsulated by secreted bone matrix and are suggested to coordinate the location of bone formation or resorption [12]. The packed osteons is the bone matrix, surrounding and protecting the medullary cavity of the diaphysis, containing bone marrow, with a thin connective tissue membrane separating both. The hematopoietic lineage in the bone marrow is responsible for pre-osteoclastogenesis [14, 15]. The macrophage colony-stimulating factor (M-CSF) stimulates the progenitor bone marrow cell for differentiation into a pre-osteoclast, initiating the expression of the receptor activator of NF-κB (RANK) receptor [16, 17]. The osteoblasts express the opposite part of the RANK receptor, necessary for activation, the RANK ligand (RANKL). Upon activation of RANK by RANKL the osteoblasts ensure that several activated pre-osteoclasts fuse together, forming a larger multinucleated mature osteoclast [16]. A mature osteoclast is a specialized macrophage with multiple mitochondria and lysosomes, prepared for bone degradation [14, 15]. In addition, the cell–cell fusion process of pre-osteoclasts forming a mature osteoclast has a checkpoint, the stromal cells, which have the ability to interfere by secretion of Osteoprotegerin (OPG). This is a decoy receptor able to bind excessive levels of RANKL, preventing over-population of osteoclasts [9, 16, 18, 19]. Subsequently, the degradation of bone is initiated after maturation of osteoclasts and their allocation to the site-of-destruction, where they form a closed space, the resorption lacuna. Activation of H^+-ATPase proton pump and Cl/HCO_3 exchanger by osteoclasts follows, in combination with the secretion of lysosomal enzymes and active protease Cathepsin K into the lacuna [15]. The net effect of this cascade is an acidic environment of pH + 4.5 to degrade the nearby bone cells [9, 15]. This triad of RANK/RANKL/OPG that regulates osteoclast activation is an important process in healthy bone physiology and plays an important role during bone cancer pain development [16–20]. Finally, At the level where the diaphysis reaches the proximal epiphysis, the medullary cavity is more spongy-like and is called trabecular or cancellous bone. Both epiphyses are composed primarily of spongy bone and a small quantity of compact bone, surrounded by cartilage [7].

Nociceptors are necessary to let the brain perceive CIBP, however, very little is known regarding the innervation of bone with sensory nerve fibers. Immunoreactivity studies have shown that sensory neurons are present in periosteum, cambium, bone matrix, Haversian canals and in bone marrow in the medullary cavity, and no detection was found in the articular cartilage of the epiphysis [21–29]. The density (nerves per unit area) of sensory fibers is largest in the periosteum, followed by bone marrow, mineralized bone and articular cartilage consisting in a ratio of 100:2:0.1:0, respectively [9, 10, 28]. Up to 80% of the nerve fibers innervating the bone have been shown TrkA positive [22], suggesting innervation of mostly thin myelinated Aδ-fibers and unmyelinated C-fibers [9, 10, 29, 30]. It seems that the fast conducting, highly myelinated Aβ-fibers do not contribute, or very scarcely, to the innervation of sensory neurons in the bone [29].

2.2 Epidemiology and primary vs. secondary tumors

The world health organization (WHO) report from 2014 predicted that a total of 19 million cancer cases exist globally in 2025 [18] and in 2018 a WHO press release announced that lung (2.09 million cases), breast (2.09 million cases), colorectal (1.08 million cases) and prostate (1.28 million cases) are the most common [31]. All of these, except for colorectal, follow a high pattern of bone metastasis in 60 to 84% of the cases [9, 32]. In breast and prostate cancer patients particularly, it is expected that 90% develop bone metastases [33, 34]. Additionally, there are primary bone tumors that have their origin within the bone and the most common type is an osteosarcoma with a worldwide incidence of 3.4 cases per million people per year [35]. In pediatrics it accounts for 3 to 5% of the cancers and in adults less than 1% [8]. Tumors can affect osteoblasts, resulting in osteoblastic lesions and in contrast affect osteoclasts, causing osteolytic lesions [36]. Primary bone tumors, e.g. osteosarcoma, are more osteolytic [37], prostate cancer seems more osteoblastic and breast cancer osteolytic [38]. The latter two have been observed in 1/4th of the cases to be mixed [39]. A specific group of well-known signaling proteins, the Wnt pathway, is suggested to shift tumors towards an osteoblastic phenotype as blockage showed a highly osteolytic tumor [40]. This pathway has been observed to directly enhance osteoblast differentiation and bone formation, whereas indirectly inhibits osteoclast differentiation and bone resorption by OPG production from osteoblasts and osteocytes [41].

Some cancer patients encounter bone tumors without the presence of pain. Unfortunately, 30 to 50% of the patients will experience mild to moderate pain and in advanced cancer patients 75 to 90% have life-altering pain [37, 42]. The most prevalent type of pain experienced is bone cancer pain [9, 17, 33], which patients describe as a persistent presence of a dull ache that increases in intensity over time [32]. They start noticing mechanical allodynia during normal activities, such as coughing, turning in bed or gentle limb movements [43]. Furthermore, there is incident pain, that occurs when the pain spontaneously intensifies as a result of weight-bearing or during movement. Finally, there are breakthrough events of very sharp intense pain that can happen during rest [9, 32]. These breakthrough pain episodes occur in 40 to 80% of the patients with a median of 4 episodes per day, lasting up to 30 minutes [44]. Particularly the incident and breakthrough pain events are devastating for the quality of life and are considered as most difficult pain conditions to treat [9, 33].

2.3 Mechanism of action of bone cancer pain

The Aδ-fibers are recognized to be important in acute pain, whereas C-fibers are the slower conducting sensors that account for physiological changes such as "second pain" [9]. It has been observed during chronic pain that these start sprouting and show enhanced spontaneous activity, ectopic firing, resulting in allodynia and hyperalgesia [45–48]. Important surface channels and receptors of Aδ- and C-fibers involved in nociceptive signaling are TrkA, acid sensing ion channels (ASIC), Transient receptor vanilloid-1 (TRPV1), P2X receptors, endothelin receptor (ET-1), bradykinin receptor (B_2R), prostaglandin (PGE_2) receptor, the voltage-gated sodium channels Na.v1.7–1.9 and cytokine receptors [9, 18, 29, 49].

The mechanism of CIBP in osteoblastic lesions is poorly understood and the most influential factors described are bone morphogenetic factors and endothelin-1. The mechanisms in osteolytic lesions have been better elucidated [36]. First, the infiltrating tumor cells start an interaction with the stromal cells, resulting in a cascade of different pathways, shown in **Figure 1**. A primary effect on sensory nerve fibers occurs as the secreted mediators, e.g. NGF, PGE_2, transforming growth factor-β (TGF-β), bradykinin, endothelin, cytokines (e.g. IL-1, IL-6, IL-8, IL-11 and IL-17) are ligands for the receptors and cause excitation of the nerve fibers [17, 22, 29, 50–53]. It has been shown in a rat CIBP model that IL-6 plays a pivotal

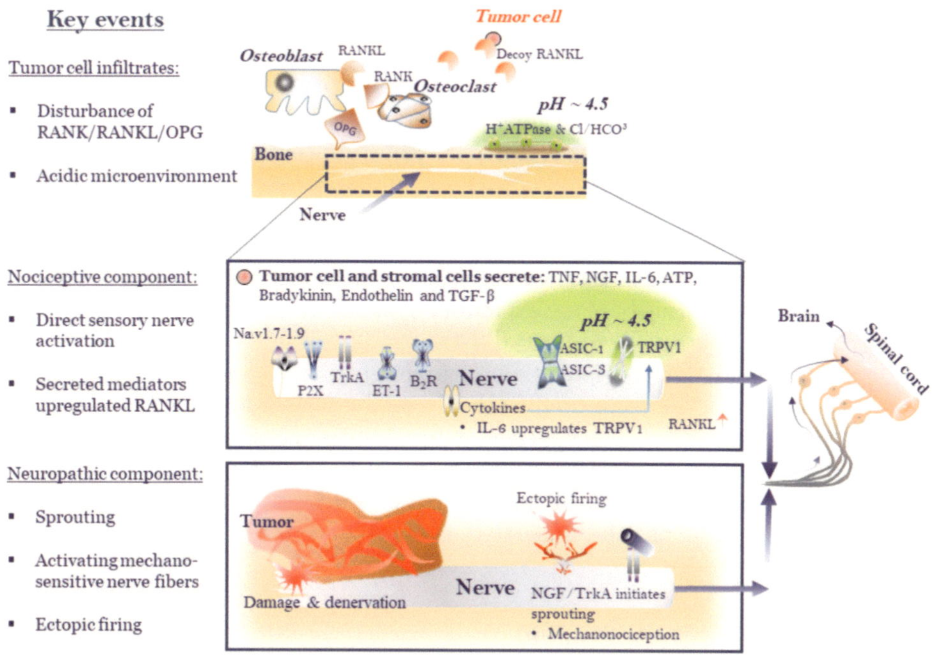

Figure 1.
The cascade of events responsible after infiltration of a tumor cell, resulting in CIBP with a nociceptive and neuropathic component. First, disturbance of the RANK/RANKL/OPG triad. Next, the nociceptive component; an acidic environment occurs, directly activating sensory nerve fibers and secreted mediators contribute to the upregulation of RANKL. In addition, the neuro-inflammatory mediator upregulates TRPV1 channels. The neuropathic component; nerves are damaged and denervate, resulting in ectopic firing and sprouting and an enlarged tumor activates mechano-sensitive nociceptors. The NGF/TrkA is pivotal in the process of sprouting and thereby for hypersensitivity. RANK = receptor activator of NF-κB, RANKL = RANK ligand, OPG = osteoprotegerin, Na.v1.7–1.9 = sodium channels, P2X = purinergic receptor, TrkA = Tromomyocin receptor kinase a, NGF = nerve growth factor, ET1 = endothelin receptor, B_2R = bradykinin receptor, ATP = Adenosinetriphosphate, IL-6 = interleukin-6, ASIC = acid-sensing ion channel, TRPV1 = transient receptor vanilloid-1, TGF-β = transforming growth factor-β, TNF = tumor growth factor.

role by sensitizing nociceptive fibers, mediating peripheral and spinal sensitization [54] by upregulation of TRPV1 receptors via JAK/PI3K signaling in dorsal root ganglia neurons [55]. In addition, PGE_2, TGF-β, IL-1, IL-6, IL-8, IL-11 and IL-17 showed to be involved in a secondary effect, namely the ability to increase the expression of RANKL and decrease OPG [17, 19, 52, 56]. TGF-β is also released by the bone matrix and stimulates osteolytic bone destruction of cells close to the tumor cells [56]. The normally present OPG that serves as a peace-keeper between osteoclasts and osteoblasts is overwhelmed by the excessive amounts of RANKL, resulting in exaggerated activity of osteoclasts [19]. Consequently, osteoclastogenesis is initiated resulting in many resorption lacunae creating an acidic environment [20]. Additional pro-inflammatory cells become active, secreted cytokines bind their designated receptors and proton (H^+ & Na^+) amounts increase, lowering the pH and thereby triggering P2X7 and TRPV1 receptors, and ASICs [1, 20, 49]. The rapid Na^+ influx is associated with ASICs and a second slow current activated at pH < 6.2 is typical for TRPV1 [20]. Subsequently, tumor cells release NGF, tumor necrosis factor (TNF), IL-1 and IL-6, chemokines and endothelins which contribute to further develop an acidic environment [32]. This could be the explanation regarding the difficulty of treating CIBP [29].

Next to the nociceptive component of CIBP is the neuropathic component, caused by damage or denervation of nerves, pressure of tumors on the nerves and sprouting. The degradation of bone and the damage that occurs can activate mechanosensitive ion channels, e.g. TRPV, ASIC and P2X7 [29, 57, 58]. Activated NGF regulates the maintenance of the peripheral sensory neuron system and initiates sprouting of adjacent non-injured afferents upon injury or denervation, resulting in collateral sprouting [59, 60]. Random sprouting of sensory neurons co-expressing TrkA was shown in prostate cancer metastases [9, 48] and similar in breast cancer metastases [47]. Hypersensitivity occurs as a result of sprouting, causing sensitization of sensory nerves, which in its turn induces mechanonociception (by Aδ-fibers) [59]. Changes also have been shown to occur in the central nervous system in the spinal cord where the excitatory synaptic transmission mediated through A-δ and C-fibers was enhanced [61].

On the one hand, it is suggested that the increase in activated osteoclasts causes the development of CIBP while on the other hand the secreted mediators directly exciting sensory nerve fibers is suggested to be the primary explanation [17, 51]. Nevertheless, all these multidisciplinary factors – *neurological, oncological and immunological* – contribute to CIBP and while they are described extensively, the exact mechanism remains to be elucidated.

3. Treatment of bone cancer pain

When a patient experiences bone cancer pain, the first step of therapy is tumor eradication, i.e. via chemotherapy and radiation, unfortunately in <50% of the patients the pain levels will return to pre-treatment levels [62]. Radiotherapy, described as the golden standard palliative therapy, shows full pain relief in 25% of treated patients, however, only after a month [29]. Different radiotherapy protocols showed a single radiotherapy fraction (8Gy) provides equal pain palliation compared to multiple fractions (30 or 20 Gy in 10 or 5 fractions, respectively) [63]. Low fractionated radiotherapy also caused a higher incidence of pathological fractions at site of irradiation [1]. Chemotherapy is an option for the treatment of CIBP when the tumor histology is more nociceptive, the patient did not previously receive chemotherapy and when the tumor is chemosensitive [64]. However, oxaliplatin and paclitaxel are used for animal models of induced-neuropathy to investigate hypersensitivity [65, 66].

3.1 Bisphosphonates

Bisphosphonates are agents that are often used to treat pain as a symptom [67]. They act by inhibiting farnesyl diphosphate synthase in phagocytic cells, e.g. osteoclasts, macrophages and microglia, thereby decrease extracellular acidification and consequently reduce ASIC- and TRPV1-mediated activation of nociceptive primary afferents located in bone [67]. Other effects of bisphosphonates unrelated to farnesyl diphosphate synthase inhibition that have been suggested are interactions with purinergic receptors, e.g. P2X7. The bisphosphonate zoledronate exerted an analgesic effects in rat CIBP models [68]. It is the most widely used bisphosphonate, also observed to significantly reduce CIBP in clinical practice for breast cancer metastases [69], being 100 to 1000 times more effective than pamidronate [70]. Furthermore, anti-inflammatory effects have been indicated where alendronate inhibited TNF-α, IL-1, IL-6 and NGF [67].

3.2 Monoclonal antibody therapy

Monoclonal antibody therapies have the ability to interfere with tumor-induced processes, e.g. RANK/RANKL, NGF/TrkA, and inhibit or avoid cytotoxic T lymphocyte [71]. A hand full of these therapies have been FDA approved for cancer therapy and a small amount has been tested in breast, prostate or lung cancer metastases [71]. Tanezumab is a monoclonal antibody interfering with NGF/TrkA and has been described unbeneficial in one CIBP study [72], however, has also been shown to attenuate late stage cancer pain [73]. Denosumab is another monoclonal antibody and acts by interfering with the interaction between RANK/RANKL, capturing RANKL, resulting in osteoclast inactivation [74]. Denosumab has been tested as treatment in breast cancer metastases and while it showed a good activity profile for delaying or preventing skeletal related events, no direct relief of pain has been described. Nevertheless, the delay and/or prevention of skeletal related events would have an indirect pain-impairing potential as such events are associated with pain and increased morbidity [75]. Denosumab did show superiority concerning first on-study skeletal-related events compared to zoledronate [76]. Similar outcomes were found by a meta-analysis of 4 RCTs between denosumab and zoledronate [77]. Regarding the dosing, a study showed no difference between 4-weekly and 12-weekly administration for denosumab and the two bisphosphonates zoledronate and pamidronate, suggesting that incorporating 12-weekly dosing could benefit patients [78]. Denosumab seems to be the only antibody therapy so far that is approved for direct treatment of skeletal-related events with bone metastases from solid tumors and giant cell tumors of the bone [71]. Ipilimumab is an antibody that activates the immune system, specifically, inhibits an inhibitory mechanism of cytotoxic T lymphocytes. It was tested in metastatic prostate cancer in combination with radiotherapy and suggested clinical antitumor activity [79]. Nivolumab therapy was recently tested in lung cancer metastases into the bone and showed that 40% of the treated patients had osteosclerotic change on CT scans, indicating successful treatment of bone lesions [80]. The small amount of monoclonal antibodies used for bone metastases often have skeletal related events as indication of efficacy but lack bone cancer pain as direct outcome measure. Currently there are no recorded monoclonal antibodies specifically targeting CIBP.

3.3 Analgesics: NSAIDs and opioids

Available options for the direct treatment of CIBP are analgesics. The WHO has established a 3-step ladder as a guideline for analgesic prescription in 1986 and revised the version in 1996 with a quick guide to opioid availability [81]. Afterwards, the stigma on opioid prescription was broken and received acceptance as treatment for (chronic) pain conditions [82–84]. The 3-step ladder starts with non-opioids (Step 1) for mild pain, weak opioids ± non-opioids and adjuvants for mild to moderate pain (Step 2), and strong opioids ± non-opioids and adjuvants for moderate to severe pain (Step 3) [85].

First in line are NSAIDs that inhibit the enzyme cyclooxygenase-2 (COX-2), responsible for PGE synthesis [64]. A challenge with NSAIDs is that they reach a ceiling effect in analgesic efficacy [81, 86]. Increasing the doses does not result in increased efficacy, conversely, side effects worsen, further impairing the quality of life of patients [86, 87]. Second in line are weak opioids, e.g. codeine, tapentadol or tramadol, in combination with adjuvants, indicating proven analgesic efficacy in bone cancer pain [88]. There are three classical opioid receptors, e.g. the μ-, δ- and κ-opioid receptors (MOP, DOP and KOP receptor, respectively) and the later discovered Nocicpetin/OrphaninFQ opioid peptide (NOP) receptor [89]. These receptors are G-protein coupled receptors and upon activation initiate an intracellular cascade resulting in 1) the inhibition of adenylate cyclase (responsible for cAMP production), 2) opening of inwardly rectifying K^+ channels and

3) closing of voltage-gated Ca^{2+} channels [89]. Caution must be exercised with weak opioids as the rate of metabolism by Cytochrome P450 enzymes defines analgesic efficacy and side effects. In addition, codeine seemed effective for only 1 month until strong opioids were necessary for adequate analgesia [90, 91]. A randomized RCT trial showed significant impairment of cancer pain by low-dose morphine compared with weak opioids, with similar tolerability and an earlier effect, suggesting low-dose morphine can be used [90, 92]. This forwards the therapy option towards Step 3 and to date, the first choice to treat moderate to severe pain with strong opioids remains morphine [90, 93]. MOP receptor drugs have shown superior analgesic efficacy and have been used for centuries as they seem to be the most potent analgesics [94]. Available options for administration are oral and transdermal, showing similar efficacy, and advocated is the use of epidural or intrathecal pumps if relief is inadequate [90]. Concerning side effects of MOP receptor drugs are addiction and dependency. The opioid crisis is prove and accounted for 33.000 deaths per year in the US by opioid misuse [94–96]. In addition, cancer survivors showed higher opioid prescription compared to controls [97]. The total estimated economic burden due to opioid addiction, dependency, abuse and overdose is $78.5 billion, from which $28.9 billion is due to increased health care and abuse treatment [98]. Furthermore, analgesic efficacy of MOP receptor compounds is affected by long term opioid treatment as tolerance develops over time [99, 100]. This is inevitable in cancer patients since high doses are required for pain management [101]. The mechanism that contributes pre-synaptically to tolerance remains to be elucidated but TRPV1 receptor upregulation in spinal cord and dorsal root ganglions has been shown to accompany tolerance [99, 100].

Challenging is to find analgesics with a similar potency and efficacy compared to MOP receptors, without dependency and addiction. Targeting the DOP and KOP receptor showed efficacious pain relief with a lower abuse potential, making them promising targets for treating pain [102]. Specifically for CIBP, both DOP and KOP receptor agonists showed pain attenuation in animal models of CIBP [103, 104]. It has been shown that a selective KOP receptor agonist blocked pain without altering bone loss, tumor size or cancer cell proliferation [105]. Additionally, a DOP receptor agonist showed equal analgesic efficacy and 4.5-fold potency compared to morphine in a mouse CIBP model [106]. Despite potential analgesic efficacy, MOP receptor agonists remain the clinical mainstay [107, 108]. Interest in the NOP receptor increased after the discovery of similar, yet distinct features compared to the classical opioids [109]. The effects of classical opioids are immediately blocked by naloxone and independently of administration location, they attenuate pain. The analgesic NOP receptor effect remains after naloxone and interestingly, spinal or peripheral activation exerts anti-nociceptive effects, while supra-spinally it acts pro-nociceptive [85, 109]. Following these discoveries, the NOP receptor showed anti-rewarding and anti-abuse effects in rodents [85, 110–113]. Furthermore, NOP receptor expressing Chinese Hamster Ovary cells showed rapid internalization after activation and a quick recycle process to reactivate receptors occurred at the membrane, potentially reducing the development of tolerance. However, compensatory mechanisms that remain to be elucidated may be overlooked [114]. The NOP receptor has been specifically used to target CIBP and both the endogenous ligand Nociceptin and a synthetic selective NOP receptor agonist (Ro65–6570) showed significant analgesia [85]. Furthermore, NOP receptor activation downregulates IL-6 production [115] and is suggested to inhibit T cell proliferation [116]. Altogether, the anti-rewarding and anti-abuse effects, cytokine production involvement and selective attenuation of CIBP, makes the NOP receptor an interesting target.

3.4 Primary vs. secondary tumor treatment

Differences should be kept in mind when treating tumors, nevertheless, anti-NGF antibody therapy has been observed to relief early and late stage CIBP in a primary bone tumor model and a metastatic-like prostate bone cancer model [37]. In addition, zoledronate has been shown effective in reducing the risk of skeletal related events in multiple myeloma, prostate and breast cancer bone metastasis [117]. Denosumab indicated superiority to zoledronate in preventing skeletal related events in bone metastasis compared to solid tumors, suggesting a treatment option for bone metastasis [118]. Primary bone tumors are characterized by high complexity and heterogeneity in genomic alterations and are therefore challenging for developing targeted therapeutic strategies [41] which also may not satisfactorily address their metastatic counterparts [119].

3.5 Non-pharmacological interventional treatment

The WHO analgesic ladder has proven to be very helpful, nevertheless, an estimated 12% of patients remains inadequately treated for CIBP [120]. Therefore, a fourth step has been proposed that includes interventional approaches to provide a minimal acceptable quality of life [120–122]. As such, percutaneous neurolysis is performed using chemical agents or thermal energy upon celiac plexus, splanchnic nerve, superior hypogastric plexus, brachial plexus and epidural and intrathecal [120, 122]. Commonly used neurolytic agents are absolute alcohol (diluted to 50% alcohol), 6% aqueous phenol and 6% phenol in glycerine [120].

Finally, PET/CT allows the distinction between osteolytic and osteoblastic lesions and thereby detect more subtle responses to treatment regimens [123]. Using CT in the surgical planning could shift the priority of debulking dense bone to surgical reconstruction when bone metastasis is more osteolytic instead of osteoblastic [39].

4. Bone cancer pain: research techniques

The current treatments are often targeted against pain as a symptom and therapy options specifically for CIBP are rare. To elucidate the complex mechanism of action of CIBP and develop novel analgesics, further research is warranted. As such, *in vitro* techniques are an option, however, these capture a minor aspect of the complexity and as long as no technique exists that simulates this, *in vivo* research is inevitable. Nevertheless, it should be conducted highly ethically and additional regulations were established in 2009 to maintain the animals' welfare by following 3R's (Reduction, Refinement and Replacement) [124]. Furthermore, to test a nociceptive phenotype in a comfortable manner, more focus is towards animals' ethological and evolutionary preserved behavior. Finally, the *in vivo* model that is used should represent the disease and clinical symptoms as close as possible. Three criteria are important in the validation of animal models [125], 1) Face validity: the biology and symptoms as seen in humans are similar in the animal model, 2) Predictive validity: if the clinical intervention has an equal response in the animal model and 3) Construct validity: the target one is investigating exerts the same biological processes in both organisms, e.g. opioid receptors are responsible for pain relief.

4.1 *In Vivo* models for bone cancer pain

At start, to reflect metastases as closely as possible, cancer cells were injected either intravenously or intra-cardially. Face validity is achieved but uncontrolled

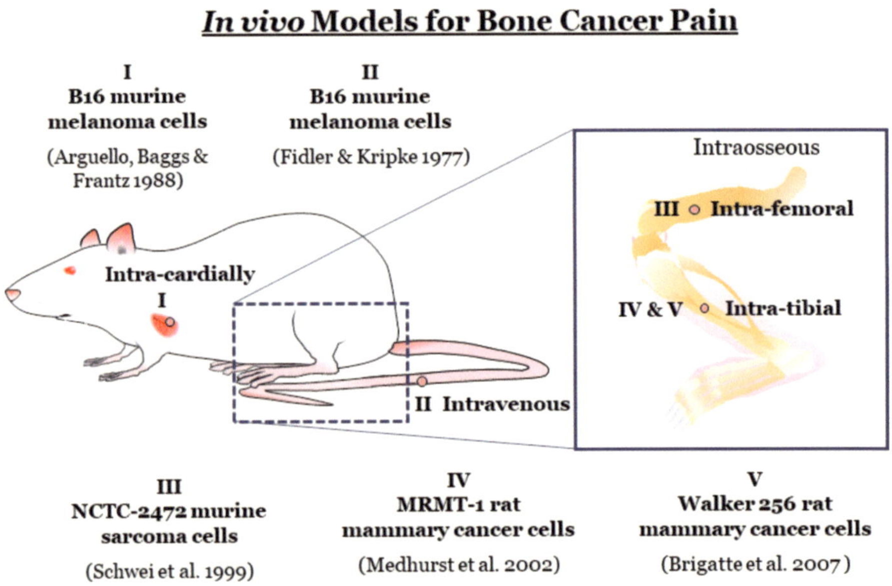

Figure 2.
A representation of the different in vivo models to study cancer induced bone pain.

growth of tumors occurs [32, 126, 127]. Next came the technique of injecting osteosarcoma-derived mesenchymal cells (NCTC-2472) directly into the long bones of mice [128]. This technique indicates good face and predictive validity, resulting in a controlled late-phase CIBP model, reflecting the clinical course with a comparable responsiveness to systemic opioid treatment [32, 128]. Finally, construct validity had been optimized using syngeneic cell lines (originating from the same species). The first example was rat mammary gland carcinoma cells (MRMT-1 cell line) inoculation into the tibia of rats [129]. The main characteristics after inoculation of cancer cells are: development of allodynia and hyperalgesia, progressive tumor growth, profound destruction and rebuilding of bone and no external tumor growth into other organs. In addition, upregulation of TNF-α, Interferon- γ (IFN-γ), IL-1β, IL-4, IL-10 and IL-6 occurs in tumor-bearing animals [49, 130]. Fine-tuning occurred with another rat breast cancer cell line (Walker 256 cells) inoculated into the tibia [131]. This model has been reviewed extensively and develops spontaneous pain, hyperalgesia, allodynia as well as ambulatory pain, indicates progressive tumor growth with osteolysis and no external growth, including upregulation of IL-1β, NGF, PGE_2, IL-6 and TNFα [132]. This model has been subjected to a detailed pharmacological profiling using standard analgesic drugs for CIBP in a clinical setting and is suggested to be one of the most suitable preclinical models for novel compound identification and assessment [132, 133]. No study has been conducted comparing the Walker 256 model with the MRMT-1 model (**Figure 2**).

5. Conclusion

Cancer-induced bone pain (CIBP) causes life-altering pain in 75 to 90% of the advanced stage cancer patients. The movement-induced incident and breakthrough events cause a severe impairment of the quality of life of patients and explain the difficulty to treat this unique type of pain. There remains a high unmet medical need for CIBP treatment since around one-third of the advanced cancer patients is still undertreated [90]. Apparent from the mechanism of actions is that CIBP concerns distinct processes and could be treated by pharmacological and non-pharmacological options. Strategies are to combine therapies, such as co-administration of zoledronate via a new innovative nano-agent with cisplatin and alendronate for breast cancer metastases and bone resorption, showing remarkable inhibition of tumor cell proliferation, osteoclast activation and bone pain relief [134]. Mixed ligands are another strategy, such as Cebranopadol, a mixed NOP/Opioid receptor ligand, indicating antinociceptive and antihypersensitive effects in a rat model of CIBP [135]. A meta-analysis comparing the efficacy of NSAID, opioids and monoclonal NGF antibodies indicate the latter provide superior pain relief, noteworthy is that this was in osteoarthritis [136]. As new strategies are arising, bisphosphonates and denosumab are the first-line therapies for bone metastases [38] and continuing research is warranted to elucidate the CIBP mechanism for identifying novel analgesic compounds.

Author details

Sonny Hermanus Johannes Sliepen
Dutch Independent Researcher, Hamburg, Germany

*Address all correspondence to: sonny.sliepen@gmail.com

References

[1] Zajączkowska, R., et al., *Bone Pain in Cancer Patients: Mechanisms and Current Treatment.* International journal of molecular sciences, 2019. **20**(23): p. 6047 DOI: 10.3390/ijms20236047.

[2] Kandel, E.R., Schwartz, J.H., Jessell, T.M., *Principles of Neural Science*. 4th ed, ed. J.B.a.H. Lebowitz. 2000, United States of America: McGraw-Hill Companies, Inc. 411-492

[3] Latremoliere, A. and C.J. Woolf, *Central sensitization: a generator of pain hypersensitivity by central neural plasticity.* J Pain, 2009. **10**(9): p. 895-926 DOI: 10.1016/j.jpain.2009.06.012.

[4] Treede, R.-D., et al., *Chronic pain as a symptom or a disease: the IASP Classification of Chronic Pain for the International Classification of Diseases (ICD-11).* PAIN, 2019. **160**(1): p. 19-27 DOI: 10.1097/j.pain.0000000000001384.

[5] Loeser, J.D. and R.D. Treede, *The Kyoto protocol of IASP Basic Pain Terminology.* Pain, 2008. **137**(3): p. 473-7 DOI: 10.1016/j.pain.2008.04.025.

[6] Muley, M.M., E. Krustev, and J.J. McDougall, *Preclinical Assessment of Inflammatory Pain.* CNS Neurosci Ther, 2016. **22**(2): p. 88-101 DOI: 10.1111/cns.12486.

[7] Buckwalter, J.A., et al., *Bone biology. I: Structure, blood supply, cells, matrix, and mineralization.* Instr Course Lect, 1996. **45**: p. 371-86.

[8] Mirabello, L., R.J. Troisi, and S.A. Savage, *International osteosarcoma incidence patterns in children and adolescents, middle ages and elderly persons.* Int J Cancer, 2009. **125**(1): p. 229-34 DOI: 10.1002/ijc.24320.

[9] Mantyh, P.W., *Bone cancer pain: from mechanism to therapy.* Curr Opin Support Palliat Care, 2014. **8**(2): p. 83-90 DOI: 10.1097/SPC.0000000000000048.

[10] Mantyh, P.W., *Mechanisms that drive bone pain across the lifespan.* Br J Clin Pharmacol, 2018 DOI: 10.1111/bcp.13801.

[11] Augustin, G., A. Antabak, and S. Davila, *The periosteum. Part 1: Anatomy, histology and molecular biology.* Injury, 2007. **38**(10): p. 1115-30 DOI: 10.1016/j.injury.2007.05.017.

[12] Caetano-Lopes, J., H. Canhao, and J.E. Fonseca, *Osteoblasts and bone formation.* Acta Reumatol Port, 2007. **32**(2): p. 103-10.

[13] Delgado-Calle, J. and T. Bellido, *Osteocytes and Skeletal Pathophysiology.* Curr Mol Biol Rep, 2015. **1**(4): p. 157-167 DOI: 10.1007/s40610-015-0026-y.

[14] Horowitz, M.C., et al., *B cells and osteoblast and osteoclast development.* Immunol Rev, 2005. **208**: p. 141-53 DOI: 10.1111/j.0105-2896.2005.00328.x.

[15] Teitelbaum, S.L., *Bone resorption by osteoclasts.* Science, 2000. **289**(5484): p. 1504-8.

[16] Sisay, M., G. Mengistu, and D. Edessa, *The RANK/RANKL/OPG system in tumorigenesis and metastasis of cancer stem cell: potential targets for anticancer therapy.* Onco Targets Ther, 2017. **10**: p. 3801-3810 DOI: 10.2147/OTT.S135867.

[17] Dougall, W.C. and M. Chaisson, *The RANK/RANKL/OPG triad in cancer-induced bone diseases.* Cancer Metastasis Rev, 2006. **25**(4): p. 541-9 DOI: 10.1007/s10555-006-9021-3.

[18] Zhu, X.C., et al., *Advances in cancer pain from bone metastasis.* Drug Des Devel Ther, 2015. **9**: p. 4239-45 DOI: 10.2147/DDDT.S87568.

[19] Rao, S., et al., *RANKL and RANK: From Mammalian Physiology to Cancer Treatment.* Trends Cell Biol, 2018. **28**(3): p. 213-223 DOI: 10.1016/j.tcb.2017.11.001.

[20] Yoneda, T., et al., *Acidic microenvironment and bone pain in cancer-colonized bone.* Bonekey Rep, 2015. **4**: p. 690 DOI: 10.1038/bonekey.2015.58.

[21] Mach, D.B., et al., *Origins of skeletal pain: sensory and sympathetic innervation of the mouse femur.* Neuroscience, 2002. **113**(1): p. 155-66 DOI: 10.1016/s0306-4522(02)00165-3.

[22] Chartier, S.R., et al., *The Changing Sensory and Sympathetic Innervation of the Young, Adult and Aging Mouse Femur.* Neuroscience, 2018. **387**: p. 178-190 DOI: 10.1016/j.neuroscience.2018.01.047.

[23] Sayilekshmy, M., et al., *Innervation is higher above Bone Remodeling Surfaces and in Cortical Pores in Human Bone: Lessons from patients with primary hyperparathyroidism.* Sci Rep, 2019. **9**(1): p. 5361 DOI: 10.1038/s41598-019-41779-w.

[24] Grönblad, M., et al., *Innervation of human bone periosteum by peptidergic nerves.* Anat Rec, 1984. **209**(3): p. 297-9 DOI: 10.1002/ar.1092090306.

[25] Ivanusic, J.J., *Size, neurochemistry, and segmental distribution of sensory neurons innervating the rat tibia.* J Comp Neurol, 2009. **517**(3): p. 276-83 DOI: 10.1002/cne.22160.

[26] Irie, K., et al., *Calcitonin gene-related peptide (CGRP)-containing nerve fibers in bone tissue and their involvement in bone remodeling.* Microsc Res Tech, 2002. **58**(2): p. 85-90 DOI: 10.1002/jemt.10122.

[27] Hukkanen, M., et al., *Innervation of bone from healthy and arthritic rats by substance P and calcitonin gene related peptide containing sensory fibers.* J Rheumatol, 1992. **19**(8): p. 1252-9.

[28] Castañeda-Corral, G., et al., *The majority of myelinated and unmyelinated sensory nerve fibers that innervate bone express the tropomyosin receptor kinase A.* Neuroscience, 2011. **178**: p. 196-207 DOI: 10.1016/j.neuroscience.2011.01.039.

[29] Hua, B., et al., *New insights of nociceptor sensitization in bone cancer pain.* Expert Opin Ther Targets, 2015. **19**(2): p. 227-43 DOI: 10.1517/14728222.2014.980815.

[30] Nencini, S., et al., *Mechanisms of nerve growth factor signaling in bone nociceptors and in an animal model of inflammatory bone pain.* Mol Pain, 2017. **13**: p. 1744806917697011 DOI: 10.1177/1744806917697011.

[31] WHO. *Cancer - Key facts [Internet].* 2018; Available from: https://www.who.int/news-room/fact-sheets/detail/cancer [Accessed: 2020 2020-12-22].

[32] Urch, C., *The pathophysiology of cancer-induced bone pain: current understanding.* Palliat Med, 2004. **18**(4): p. 267-74 DOI: 10.1191/0269216304pm887ra.

[33] Lucchesi, M., et al., *Developing drugs in cancer-related bone pain.* Crit Rev Oncol Hematol, 2017. **119**: p. 66-74 DOI: 10.1016/j.critrevonc.2017.08.005.

[34] Coleman, R.E., *Clinical features of metastatic bone disease and risk of skeletal morbidity.* Clin Cancer Res, 2006. **12**(20 Pt 2): p. 6243s–6249s DOI: 10.1158/1078-0432.CCR-06-0931.

[35] Misaghi, A., et al., *Osteosarcoma: a comprehensive review.* SICOT J, 2018. **4**: p. 12 DOI: 10.1051/sicotj/2017028.

[36] Schmid-Alliana, A., et al., *Understanding the Progression of Bone*

Metastases to Identify Novel Therapeutic Targets. International journal of molecular sciences, 2018. **19**(1): p. 148 DOI: 10.3390/ijms19010148.

[37] Halvorson, K.G., et al., *Similarities and differences in tumor growth, skeletal remodeling and pain in an osteolytic and osteoblastic model of bone cancer.* Clin J Pain, 2006. **22**(7): p. 587-600 DOI: 10.1097/01.ajp.0000210902.67849.e6.

[38] He, F. and Y. Matsumoto, *Basic and clinical associations between bone and cancer.* Immunol Med, 2020. **43**(3): p. 103-106 DOI: 10.1080/25785826.2020.1754084.

[39] Reddington, J.A., et al., *Imaging characteristic analysis of metastatic spine lesions from breast, prostate, lung, and renal cell carcinomas for surgical planning: Osteolytic versus osteoblastic.* Surg Neurol Int, 2016. **7**(Suppl 13): p. S361-5 DOI: 10.4103/2152-7806.182549.

[40] Hall, C.L., et al., *Prostate cancer cells promote osteoblastic bone metastases through Wnts.* Cancer Res, 2005. **65**(17): p. 7554-60 DOI: 10.1158/0008-5472.Can-05-1317.

[41] Danieau, G., et al., *New Insights about the Wnt/β-Catenin Signaling Pathway in Primary Bone Tumors and Their Microenvironment: A Promising Target to Develop Therapeutic Strategies?* International journal of molecular sciences, 2019. **20**(15): p. 3751 DOI: 10.3390/ijms20153751.

[42] Zhao, C., et al., *Analgesic effects of a soy-containing diet in three murine bone cancer pain models.* J Pain, 2004. **5**(2): p. 104-10 DOI: 10.1016/j.jpain.2003.12.001.

[43] Clohisy, D.R. and P.W. Mantyh, *Bone cancer pain.* Cancer, 2003. **97**(3 Suppl): p. 866-73 DOI: 10.1002/cncr.11144.

[44] Davis, M.P., et al., *Controversies in pharmacotherapy of pain management.* Lancet Oncol, 2005. **6**(9): p. 696-704 DOI: 10.1016/S1470-2045(05)70317-X.

[45] Carlton, S.M., et al., *Peripheral and central sensitization in remote spinal cord regions contribute to central neuropathic pain after spinal cord injury.* Pain, 2009. **147**(1-3): p. 265-76 DOI: 10.1016/j.pain.2009.09.030.

[46] Walters, E.T., *Nociceptors as chronic drivers of pain and hyperreflexia after spinal cord injury: an adaptive-maladaptive hyperfunctional state hypothesis.* Front Physiol, 2012. **3**: p. 309 DOI: 10.3389/fphys.2012.00309.

[47] Bloom, A.P., et al., *Breast cancer-induced bone remodeling, skeletal pain, and sprouting of sensory nerve fibers.* J Pain, 2011. **12**(6): p. 698-711 DOI: 10.1016/j.jpain.2010.12.016.

[48] Jimenez-Andrade, J.M., et al., *Pathological sprouting of adult nociceptors in chronic prostate cancer-induced bone pain.* J Neurosci, 2010. **30**(44): p. 14649-56 DOI: 10.1523/JNEUROSCI.3300-10.2010.

[49] Lozano-Ondoua, A.N., A.M. Symons-Liguori, and T.W. Vanderah, *Cancer-induced bone pain: Mechanisms and models.* Neurosci Lett, 2013. **557 Pt A**: p. 52-9 DOI: 10.1016/j.neulet.2013.08.003.

[50] Brown, J.M., et al., *Osteoprotegerin and rank ligand expression in prostate cancer.* Urology, 2001. **57**(4): p. 611-6.

[51] Milgrom, D.P., et al., *Bone Pain and Muscle Weakness in Cancer Patients.* Curr Osteoporos Rep, 2017. **15**(2): p. 76-87 DOI: 10.1007/s11914-017-0354-3.

[52] Zhang, J., et al., *In vivo real-time imaging of TGF-beta-induced transcriptional activation of the RANK ligand gene promoter in intraosseous prostate cancer.* Prostate, 2004. **59**(4): p. 360-9 DOI: 10.1002/pros.20019.

[53] Bendre, M.S., et al., *Interleukin-8 stimulation of osteoclastogenesis and bone resorption is a mechanism for the increased osteolysis of metastatic bone disease.* Bone, 2003. **33**(1): p. 28-37.

[54] Remeniuk, B., et al., *Disease modifying actions of interleukin-6 blockade in a rat model of bone cancer pain.* Pain, 2018. **159**(4): p. 684-698 DOI: 10.1097/j.pain.0000000000001139.

[55] Fang, D., et al., *Interleukin-6-mediated functional upregulation of TRPV1 receptors in dorsal root ganglion neurons through the activation of JAK/PI3K signaling pathway: roles in the development of bone cancer pain in a rat model.* Pain, 2015. **156**(6): p. 1124-44 DOI: 10.1097/j.pain.0000000000000158.

[56] Chiechi, A., et al., *Role of TGF-β in breast cancer bone metastases.* Adv Biosci Biotechnol, 2013. **4**(10c): p. 15-30 DOI: 10.4236/abb.2013.410A4003.

[57] Hope, J.M., J.D. Greenlee, and M.R. King, *Mechanosensitive Ion Channels: TRPV4 and P2X7 in Disseminating Cancer Cells.* Cancer J, 2018. **24**(2): p. 84-92 DOI: 10.1097/ppo.0000000000000312.

[58] Pethő, Z., et al., *Mechanosensitive ion channels push cancer progression.* Cell Calcium, 2019. **80**: p. 79-90 DOI: 10.1016/j.ceca.2019.03.007.

[59] Jankowski, M.P. and H.R. Koerber, *Neurotrophic Factors and Nociceptor Sensitization*, in *Translational Pain Research: From Mouse to Man*, L. Kruger and A.R. Light, Editors. 2010: Boca Raton, FL.

[60] Pertens, E., et al., *Intraspinal and behavioral consequences of nerve growth factor-induced nociceptive sprouting and nerve growth factor-induced hyperalgesia compared in adult rats.* J Comp Neurol, 1999. **410**(1): p. 73-89.

[61] Yanagisawa, Y., et al., *Bone cancer induces a unique central sensitization through synaptic changes in a wide area of the spinal cord.* Mol Pain, 2010. **6**: p. 38 DOI: 10.1186/1744-8069-6-38.

[62] Clohisy, D.R. and P.W. Mantyh, *Bone cancer pain.* Clin Orthop Relat Res, 2003(415 Suppl): p. S279-88 DOI: 10.1097/01.blo.0000093059.96273.56.

[63] Niang, U., et al., *The management of painful bone metastases with biphosphonates and palliative radiotherapy: a retrospective evaluation of 372 cases.* J buon, 2009. **14**(2): p. 245-9.

[64] O'Toole, G.C. and P. Boland, *Metastatic bone cancer pain: etiology and treatment options.* Curr Pain Headache Rep, 2006. **10**(4): p. 288-92 DOI: 10.1007/s11916-006-0034-y.

[65] Micheli, L., et al., *Intrathecal administration of nociceptin/orphanin FQ receptor agonists in rats: A strategy to relieve chemotherapy-induced neuropathic hypersensitivity.* Eur J Pharmacol, 2015. **766**: p. 155-62 DOI: 10.1016/j.ejphar.2015.10.005.

[66] Griffiths, L.A., et al., *Evoked and Ongoing Pain-Like Behaviours in a Rat Model of Paclitaxel-Induced Peripheral Neuropathy.* Pain Res Manag, 2018. **2018**: p. 8217613 DOI: 10.1155/2018/8217613.

[67] Tzschentke, T.M., *Pharmacology of bisphosphonates in pain.* Br J Pharmacol, 2019 DOI: 10.1111/bph.14799.

[68] Walker, K., et al., *Disease modifying and anti-nociceptive effects of the bisphosphonate, zoledronic acid in a model of bone cancer pain.* PAIN, 2002. **100**(3): p. 219-229 DOI: 10.1016/s0304-3959(02)00040-4.

[69] Lluch, A., et al., *Zoledronic acid in the treatment of metastatic breast cancer.* Anticancer Drugs, 2014. **25**(1): p. 1-7 DOI: 10.1097/cad.0000000000000020.

[70] Yang, L. and S. Du, *Efficacy and Safety of Zoledronic Acid and Pamidronate Disodium in the Treatment of Malignant Skeletal Metastasis: A Meta-Analysis.* Medicine (Baltimore), 2015. **94**(42): p. e1822 DOI: 10.1097/md.0000000000001822.

[71] Baldo, B.A., *Monoclonal Antibodies Approved for Cancer Therapy*, in *Safety of Biologics Therapy: Monoclonal Antibodies, Cytokines, Fusion Proteins, Hormones, Enzymes, Coagulation Proteins, Vaccines, Botulinum Toxins*, B.A. Baldo, Editor. 2016, Springer International Publishing: Cham. p. 57-140.

[72] Sopata, M., et al., *Efficacy and safety of tanezumab in the treatment of pain from bone metastases.* Pain, 2015. **156**(9): p. 1703-13 DOI: 10.1097/j.pain.0000000000000211.

[73] Mantyh, W.G., et al., *Blockade of nerve sprouting and neuroma formation markedly attenuates the development of late stage cancer pain.* Neuroscience, 2010. **171**(2): p. 588-98 DOI: 10.1016/j.neuroscience.2010.08.056.

[74] Simatou, A., et al., *The Role of the RANKL/RANK Axis in the Prevention and Treatment of Breast Cancer with Immune Checkpoint Inhibitors and Anti-RANKL.* Int J Mol Sci, 2020. **21**(20) DOI: 10.3390/ijms21207570.

[75] Irelli, A., et al., *Real-life use of denosumab 120 mg every 12 weeks in prolonged treatment over 2 years of patients with breast cancer bone metastases.* J buon, 2020. **25**(4): p. 1799-1804.

[76] Stopeck, A.T., et al., *Denosumab compared with zoledronic acid for the treatment of bone metastases in patients with advanced breast cancer: a randomized, double-blind study.* J Clin Oncol, 2010. **28**(35): p. 5132-9 DOI: 10.1200/jco.2010.29.7101.

[77] Chen, J., et al., *Meta-analysis of clinical trials to assess denosumab over zoledronic acid in bone metastasis.* Int J Clin Pharm, 2020 DOI: 10.1007/s11096-020-01105-1.

[78] Clemons, M., et al., *A randomised trial of 4- versus 12-weekly administration of bone-targeted agents in patients with bone metastases from breast or castration-resistant prostate cancer.* Eur J Cancer, 2021. **142**: p. 132-140 DOI: 10.1016/j.ejca.2020.08.019.

[79] Slovin, S.F., et al., *Ipilimumab alone or in combination with radiotherapy in metastatic castration-resistant prostate cancer: results from an open-label, multicenter phase I/II study.* Ann Oncol, 2013. **24**(7): p. 1813-1821 DOI: 10.1093/annonc/mdt107.

[80] Nakata, E., et al., *Early response of bone metastases can predict tumor response in patients with non-small-cell lung cancer with bone metastases in the treatment with nivolumab.* Oncol Lett, 2020. **20**(3): p. 2977-2986 DOI: 10.3892/ol.2020.11856.

[81] Schug, S.A. and C. Chandrasena, *Pain management of the cancer patient.* Expert Opin Pharmacother, 2015. **16**(1): p. 5-15 DOI: 10.1517/14656566.2015.980723.

[82] Vargas-Schaffer, G., *Is the WHO analgesic ladder still valid? Twenty-four years of experience.* Can Fam Physician, 2010. **56**(6): p. 514-7, e202-5.

[83] Reis-Pina, P., P.G. Lawlor, and A. Barbosa, *Cancer-Related Pain Management and the Optimal Use of Opioids.* Acta Med Port, 2015. **28**(3): p. 376-81.

[84] Davis, M.P. and Z. Mehta, *Opioids and Chronic Pain: Where Is the Balance?* Curr Oncol Rep, 2016. **18**(12): p. 71 DOI: 10.1007/s11912-016-0558-1.

[85] Sliepen, S.H.J., et al., *The nociceptin/orphanin FQ receptor system as a target to alleviate cancer-induced bone pain in rats:*

Model validation and pharmacological evaluation. Br J Pharmacol, 2019 DOI: 10.1111/bph.14899.

[86] Choi, C.Y., *Chronic pain and opiate management.* Dis Mon, 2016. **62**(9): p. 334-45 DOI: 10.1016/j.disamonth.2016.05.013.

[87] Payne, R., *Limitations of NSAIDs for pain management: toxicity or lack of efficacy?* J Pain, 2000. **1**(3 Suppl): p. 14-8.

[88] Ismy, J., D.R. Emril, and Rizkidawati, *Management of cancer pain with analgetic adjuvant and weak opioid in prostate cancer bone metastases: A case series.* Ann Med Surg (Lond), 2020. **60**: p. 575-578 DOI: 10.1016/j.amsu.2020.10.070.

[89] Williams, J., *Basic Opioid Pharmacology.* Reviews in pain, 2008. **1**(2): p. 2-5 DOI: 10.1177/204946370800100202.

[90] Chapman, E.J., et al., *Practice review: Evidence-based and effective management of pain in patients with advanced cancer.* Palliat Med, 2020. **34**(4): p. 444-453 DOI: 10.1177/0269216319896955.

[91] Aroke, E.N. and J.M. Kittelsrud, *Pharmacogenetics of Postoperative Pain Management: A Review.* Aana j, 2020. **88**(3): p. 229-236.

[92] Bandieri, E., et al., *Randomized Trial of Low-Dose Morphine Versus Weak Opioids in Moderate Cancer Pain.* J Clin Oncol, 2016. **34**(5): p. 436-42 DOI: 10.1200/jco.2015.61.0733.

[93] Thota, R.S., et al., *Indian Society for Study of Pain, Cancer Pain Special Interest Group Guidelines on Pharmacological Management of Cancer Pain (Part II).* Indian J Palliat Care, 2020. **26**(2): p. 180-190 DOI: 10.4103/0973-1075.285693.

[94] Fields, H.L., *The doctor's dilemma: opiate analgesics and chronic pain.* Neuron, 2011. **69**(4): p. 591-4 DOI: 10.1016/j.neuron.2011.02.001.

[95] Shipton, E.A., E.E. Shipton, and A.J. Shipton, *A Review of the Opioid Epidemic: What Do We Do About It?* Pain Ther, 2018. **7**(1): p. 23-36 DOI: 10.1007/s40122-018-0096-7.

[96] Soelberg, C.D., et al., *The US Opioid Crisis: Current Federal and State Legal Issues.* Anesth Analg, 2017. **125**(5): p. 1675-1681 DOI: 10.1213/ANE.0000000000002403.

[97] Sutradhar, R., A. Lokku, and L. Barbera, *Cancer survivorship and opioid prescribing rates: A population-based matched cohort study among individuals with and without a history of cancer.* Cancer, 2017 DOI: 10.1002/cncr.30839.

[98] Florence, C.S., et al., *The Economic Burden of Prescription Opioid Overdose, Abuse, and Dependence in the United States, 2013.* Med Care, 2016. **54**(10): p. 901-6 DOI: 10.1097/MLR.0000000000000625.

[99] Wilson-Poe, A.R., H.J. Jeong, and C.W. Vaughan, *Chronic morphine reduces the readily releasable pool of GABA, a presynaptic mechanism of opioid tolerance.* J Physiol, 2017. **595**(20): p. 6541-6555 DOI: 10.1113/JP274157.

[100] Bao, Y., et al., *The mechanism of mu-opioid receptor (MOR)-TRPV1 crosstalk in TRPV1 activation involves morphine anti-nociception, tolerance and dependence.* Channels (Austin), 2015. **9**(5): p. 235-43 DOI: 10.1080/19336950.2015.1069450.

[101] Viet, C.T., et al., *OPRM1 Methylation Contributes to Opioid Tolerance in Cancer Patients.* J Pain, 2017. **18**(9): p. 1046-1059 DOI: 10.1016/j.jpain.2017.04.001.

[102] Vanderah, T.W., *Delta and kappa opioid receptors as suitable drug targets for pain.* Clin J Pain, 2010.

26 Suppl 10: p. S10-5 DOI: 10.1097/AJP.0b013e3181c49e3a.

[103] Otis, V., P. Sarret, and L. Gendron, *Spinal activation of delta opioid receptors alleviates cancer-related bone pain.* Neuroscience, 2011. **183**: p. 221-9 DOI: 10.1016/j.neuroscience.2011.03.052.

[104] Kim, W.M., et al., *The intrathecally administered kappa-2 opioid agonist GR89696 and interleukin-10 attenuate bone cancer-induced pain through synergistic interaction.* Anesth Analg, 2011. **113**(4): p. 934-40 DOI: 10.1213/ANE.0b013e318227824e.

[105] Edwards, K.A., et al., *A Kappa Opioid Receptor Agonist Blocks Bone Cancer Pain Without Altering Bone Loss, Tumor Size, or Cancer Cell Proliferation in a Mouse Model of Cancer-Induced Bone Pain.* J Pain, 2018. **19**(6): p. 612-625 DOI: 10.1016/j.jpain.2018.01.002.

[106] Brainin-Mattos, J., et al., *Cancer-related bone pain is attenuated by a systemically available delta-opioid receptor agonist.* Pain, 2006. **122**(1-2): p. 174-81 DOI: 10.1016/j.pain.2006.01.032.

[107] Pasternak, G.W. and Y.-X. Pan, *Mu opioids and their receptors: evolution of a concept.* Pharmacological reviews, 2013. **65**(4): p. 1257-1317 DOI: 10.1124/pr.112.007138.

[108] Azzam, A.A.H., J. McDonald, and D.G. Lambert, *Hot topics in opioid pharmacology: mixed and biased opioids.* Br J Anaesth, 2019. **122**(6): p. e136-e145 DOI: 10.1016/j.bja.2019.03.006.

[109] Schröder, W., et al., *Functional plasticity of the N/OFQ-NOP receptor system determines analgesic properties of NOP receptor agonists.* Br J Pharmacol, 2014. **171**(16): p. 3777-800 DOI: 10.1111/bph.12744.

[110] Ciccocioppo, R., et al., *Effect of nociceptin/orphanin FQ on the rewarding properties of morphine.* European Journal of Pharmacology, 2000. **404**(1): p. 153-159 DOI: https://doi.org/10.1016/S0014-2999(00)00590-2.

[111] Lin, A.P. and M.-C. Ko, *The Therapeutic Potential of Nociceptin/Orphanin FQ Receptor Agonists as Analgesics without Abuse Liability.* ACS Chemical Neuroscience, 2013. **4**(2): p. 214-224 DOI: 10.1021/cn300124f.

[112] Rutten, K., et al., *Effects of the NOP receptor agonist Ro65-6570 on the acquisition of opiate- and psychostimulant-induced conditioned place preference in rats.* European Journal of Pharmacology, 2010. **645**(1): p. 119-126 DOI: https://doi.org/10.1016/j.ejphar.2010.07.036.

[113] Rutten, K., et al., *Pharmacological blockade or genetic knockout of the NOP receptor potentiates the rewarding effect of morphine in rats.* Drug Alcohol Depend, 2011. **114**(2-3): p. 253-6 DOI: 10.1016/j.drugalcdep.2010.10.004.

[114] Spampinato, S., M. Baiula, and M. Calienni, *Agonist-regulated internalization and desensitization of the human nociceptin receptor expressed in CHO cells.* Curr Drug Targets, 2007. **8**(1): p. 137-46.

[115] Fu, X., et al., *Regulation of proinflammatory cytokines gene expression by nociceptin/orphanin FQ in the spinal cord and the cultured astrocytes.* Neuroscience, 2007. **144**(1): p. 275-85 DOI: 10.1016/j.neuroscience.2006.09.016.

[116] Waits, P.S., et al., *Nociceptin/orphanin FQ modulates human T cell function in vitro.* J Neuroimmunol, 2004. **149**(1-2): p. 110-20 DOI: 10.1016/j.jneuroim.2003.12.018.

[117] Palmieri, C., J.R. Fullarton, and J. Brown, *Comparative efficacy of bisphosphonates in metastatic breast and prostate cancer and multiple myeloma: a mixed-treatment meta-analysis.* Clin

Cancer Res, 2013. **19**(24): p. 6863-72 DOI: 10.1158/1078-0432.Ccr-13-2275.

[118] Fang, J. and Q. Xu, *Differences of osteoblastic bone metastases and osteolytic bone metastases in clinical features and molecular characteristics.* Clin Transl Oncol, 2015. **17**(3): p. 173-9 DOI: 10.1007/s12094-014-1247-x.

[119] Romano, S., et al., *Cellular and molecular background underlying the diversity in therapeutic responses between primary tumours and metastases.* Curr Med Chem, 2014. **21**(14): p. 1631-8 DOI: 10.2174/0929867311320990225.

[120] Ahmed, A., et al., *Indian Society for Study of Pain, Cancer Pain Special Interest Group Guidelines on Interventional Management for Cancer Pain.* Indian journal of palliative care, 2020. **26**(2): p. 203-209 DOI: 10.4103/0973-1075.285696.

[121] Sindhi, V. and M. Erdek, *Interventional treatments for metastatic bone cancer pain.* Pain Manag, 2019. **9**(3): p. 307-315 DOI: 10.2217/pmt-2018-0073.

[122] Filippiadis, D., S. Tutton, and A. Kelekis, *Pain management: The rising role of interventional oncology.* Diagn Interv Imaging, 2017. **98**(9): p. 627-634 DOI: 10.1016/j.diii.2017.06.015.

[123] Hsu, W.K., et al., *Characterization of osteolytic, osteoblastic, and mixed lesions in a prostate cancer mouse model using 18F-FDG and 18F-fluoride PET/CT.* J Nucl Med, 2008. **49**(3): p. 414-21 DOI: 10.2967/jnumed.107.045666.

[124] Fenwick, N., G. Griffin, and C. Gauthier, *The welfare of animals used in science: how the "Three Rs" ethic guides improvements.* The Canadian veterinary journal = La revue veterinaire canadienne, 2009. **50**(5): p. 523-530.

[125] Denayer, T., T. Stöhr, and M. van Roy, *Animal models in translational science: validation and prediction.* Elsevier Ltd. on behalf of European Society for Translational Medicine; New Horizons in Translational Medicine, 2014. **2(1), pp. 5-11**: p. 11 DOI: http://doi.org/10.1016/j.nhtm.2014.08.001

[126] Arguello, F., R.B. Baggs, and C.N. Frantz, *A murine model of experimental metastasis to bone and bone marrow.* Cancer Res, 1988. **48**(23): p. 6876-81.

[127] Fidler, I.J. and M.L. Kripke, *Metastasis results from preexisting variant cells within a malignant tumor.* Science, 1977. **197**(4306): p. 893-5.

[128] Schwei, M.J., et al., *Neurochemical and cellular reorganization of the spinal cord in a murine model of bone cancer pain.* J Neurosci, 1999. **19**(24): p. 10886-97.

[129] Medhurst, S.J., et al., *A rat model of bone cancer pain.* Pain, 2002. **96**(1-2): p. 129-40.

[130] Jiang, W., et al., *Morin Suppresses Astrocyte Activation and Regulates Cytokine Release in Bone Cancer Pain Rat Models.* Phytother Res, 2017. **31**(9): p. 1298-1304 DOI: 10.1002/ptr.5849.

[131] Brigatte, P., et al., *Walker 256 tumor-bearing rats as a model to study cancer pain.* J Pain, 2007. **8**(5): p. 412-21 DOI: 10.1016/j.jpain.2006.11.006.

[132] Shenoy, P.A., et al., *The Walker 256 Breast Cancer Cell- Induced Bone Pain Model in Rats.* Frontiers in pharmacology, 2016. **7**: p. 286-286 DOI: 10.3389/fphar.2016.00286.

[133] Shenoy, P., et al., *Optimization and In Vivo Profiling of a Refined Rat Model of Walker 256 Breast Cancer Cell-Induced Bone Pain Using Behavioral, Radiological, Histological, Immunohistochemical and Pharmacological Methods.* Front Pharmacol, 2017. **8**: p. 442 DOI: 10.3389/fphar.2017.00442.

[134] Huang, Y., et al., *Bone-seeking nanoplatform co-delivering cisplatin and zoledronate for synergistic therapy of breast cancer bone metastasis and bone resorption.* Acta Pharm Sin B, 2020. **10**(12): p. 2384-2403 DOI: 10.1016/j.apsb.2020.06.006.

[135] Linz, K., et al., *Cebranopadol: a novel potent analgesic nociceptin/orphanin FQ peptide and opioid receptor agonist.* J Pharmacol Exp Ther, 2014. **349**(3): p. 535-48 DOI: 10.1124/jpet.114.213694.

[136] Cao, Z., et al., *Targeting nerve growth factor, a new option for treatment of osteoarthritis: a network meta-analysis of comparative efficacy and safety with traditional drugs.* Aging (Albany NY), 2020. **12** DOI: 10.18632/aging.202232.

Chapter 2

Imaging of Pediatric Benign Bone Tumors

Jignesh Shah and Ankita Chauhan

Abstract

Benign bone tumors in the pediatric population can have varied clinical presentations ranging from asymptomatic to nonspecific pain, swelling, or pathological fracture. A systemic imaging approach should be utilized to evaluate for focal bone abnormalities. Radiologists must be aware of salient imaging features of pediatric benign bone tumors, as it helps to guide clinicians for further management and help decreasing patient anxiety and unnecessary medical intervention.

Keywords: Pediatric benign bone tumors, Osteoid Osteoma, Enchondroma, Non-Ossifying Fibroma

1. Introduction

Primary benign bone tumors are more common than malignancies in children. The patient's age and lesion location are two critical factors when evaluating for a bone tumor. The initial imaging modality to evaluate for a bone tumor is radiography. Radiographs confirm the presence and location of a tumor, assist in the formulation of differential diagnosis, characterize the tumor, and guide in selecting further imaging. Cross-sectional imaging is helpful for tissue characterization and for evaluating the extent of the lesions. The patient's age helps to narrow down the differential diagnosis.

2. Classification

Pediatric benign bone tumors based on the peak age of occurrence:
Child (0–10 years).
Eosinophillic Granuloma.
Simple bone cyst.
Adolescent (10–20 years).
Aneurysmal bone cyst.
Chondroblastoma.
Chondromyxoid fibroma.
Fibrous dysplasia.
Osteochondroma.
Nonossifying fibroma/fibrous cortical defect.
Osteoblastoma.
Periosteal chondroma.
Simple bone cyst.

IntechOpen

Adult:
Enchondroma.
Giant cell tumor.
Osteoblastoma.
Brown Tumor (Hyperparathyroidism).

The location of the lesion in the bone can help narrow down the differential diagnosis.

Pediatric benign bone tumors based on location in the long bones:

Epiphysis:
Chondroblastoma.
Giant cell tumor.
Metaphysis:
Aneurysmal bone cyst.
Chondromyxoid fibroma.
Enchondroma.
Nonossifying fibroma/fibrous cortical defect.
Osteochondroma.
Simple bone cyst.
Diaphysis:
Fibrous dysplasia.
Nonossifying fibroma/fibrous cortical defect.
Osteochondroma.
Osteofibrous dysplasia.
Simple bone cyst.
Aneurysmal bone cyst.
Enchondroma.

Some lesions are solitary, and others are multifocal at presentation. The following are the examples of multifocal pediatric benign bone lesions:

Brown tumors (hyperparathyroidism).
Cystic angiomatosis/lymphangiomatosis.
Enchondroma (Ollier disease, Maffucci syndrome).
Fibrous dysplasia (McCune-Albright syndrome).
Infiltrate myofibromatosis.
Langerhans cell histiocytosis.
Nonossifying fibroma (Jaffe-Campanacci Syndrome).
Osteochondroma (Diaphyseal Aclasis).
Chronic recurrent multifocal osteomyelitis (CRMO).

The following features are characteristic for nonaggressive benign bone lesions and help differentiate from aggressive malignant bone lesions:

Well-defined margins with a narrow zone of transition.
Expansion of bone from slow growth.
Smooth periosteal new bone formation.
Absence of an associated soft tissue mass.

Some benign bone tumors are adequately defined by radiographs and do not require any further imaging for diagnosis or treatment. However, most bone tumors require additional imaging; this may be in the form of CT, MRI, scintigraphy, PET scanning, and rarely ultrasound. The choice of imaging for a given tumor depends on the differential diagnostic considerations, possible treatment options, and whether the lesion is aggressive or nonaggressive.

Classification of pediatric bone tumors according to matrix or tissue type:

Cystic lesions: Unicameral (simple) bone cyst, aneurysmal bone cyst.

Osteoid matrix lesions: Enostosis, osteoma, osteoid osteoma, osteoblastoma.

Chondroid matrix: Enchondroma, chondroblastoma, chondromyxoid fibroma, osteochondroma, juxtacortical chondroma.

Fibro-osseous lesions: Nonossifying fibroma, fibrous dysplasia, osteofibrous dysplasia.

Fat containing lesions: Lipoma.

Vascular malformations: Hemangioma.

Giant cell tumors: Giant cell tumor.

Others: Langerhans cell histiocytosis.

3. Primary benign bone tumors by tissue type

Cystic bone lesions:

1. Simple bone cyst:

A simple bone cyst is also called a solitary cyst or unicameral bone cyst (UBC). A simple bone cyst is a common benign nonneoplastic lucent bony lesion mainly seen in childhood and typically asymptomatic. Approximately 85% of unicameral bone cysts occur in children and adolescents [1]. There is 2–3:1 male predominance [2]. During the active phase, the cyst increases in size and remains close to the physis. The latent phase cysts are found farther from the physis and usually do not continue to grow. Cysts may appear to migrate into diaphysis, but actually, it is the growth plate that migrates away from the cyst. The lesions are usually asymptomatic and found incidentally, although the adjacent joint's pain, swelling, and stiffness can also occur. The most frequent complication is a pathologic fracture, and this is usually the cause of presentation. 75% of patients come in with a pathologic fracture [3]. Pathologically, the cysts contain clear serosanguineous fluid surrounded by fibrous membranous lining. The proximal humerus is the most common location (in 50–60% of cases) [4]. The second most common location is the proximal femur.

On radiography, bone cysts are located centrally in the medullary cavity within the metaphysis. Most cysts are less than 3 cm in short-axis diameter but may be much larger in the long axis. The cyst wall is well-defined and sclerotic; the overlying cortex is thinned, and the lesion may be mildly expansile (**Figures 1A, 2A**). Following a fracture, a fragment of bone may be seen dependently within the cyst, called a fallen fragment sign, considered pathognomonic for a simple bone cyst [5] (**Figure 3A**).

Computed Tomography (CT) scan and Magnetic Resonance Imaging (MRI) can help exclude other entities that can potentially mimic a simple bone cyst such as an intraosseous lipoma, fibrous dysplasia, eosinophilic granuloma, giant cell tumor, nonossifying fibroma, or aneurysmal bone cyst. The CT scan helps to delineate the cyst and confirms a fallen fragment. MRI confirms the cystic nature of the lesion. The fluid contents are low signal on T1 and high signal on T2-weighted imaging (**Figure 1B** and **C**). In contrast, the cyst lining enhances, but the contents do not (**Figures 1D, 2C**). Occasionally, when presenting with intralesional hemorrhage from fracture, fluid–fluid levels may be seen representing internal degraded blood products. The internal hemorrhage may evolve into septations that can be demonstrated on MRI (**Figure 2B**).

On scintigraphy, the unicameral bone cyst appears as a focus of photopenia (cold spot). It may have increased uptake peripherally, and a photopenic center sometimes referred to as a doughnut sign. However, a pathologic fracture would cause an increased radioisotope activity.

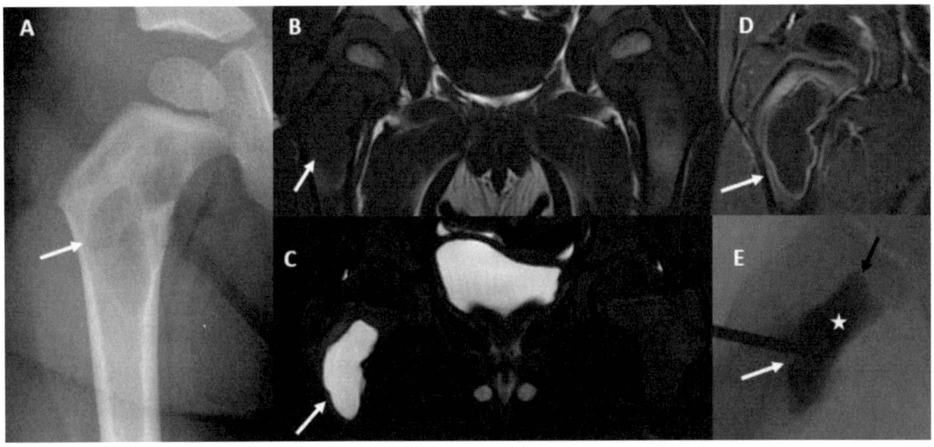

Figure 1.
Simple Bone Cyst: Frontal radiograph of the right femur demonstrates a well-circumscribed, lytic, proximal metadiaphyseal lesion (white arrow) with a narrow zone of transition and represents a simple bone cyst (A). There is no fracture. On the coronal MR sequences (B–D), the simple bone cyst (white arrows) shows an intermediate signal on T1-weighted sequence (B), a homogeneous increased signal on T2-weighted imaging (C), and peripheral rim enhancement on the post-contrast T1-weighted fat-saturated imaging (D). A simple bone cyst is treated by bone grafting. Fluoroscopic spot image of the right femur (E) confirms that the osteolytic lesion is cemented by the bone graft material (white asterisk).

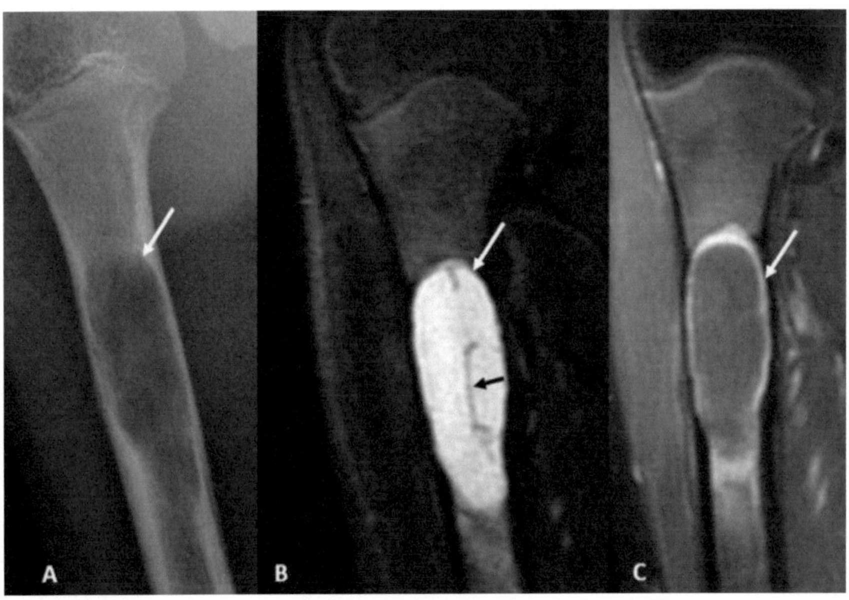

Figure 2.
Simple Bone Cyst: Frontal radiograph of the right humerus (A) demonstrates an expansile circumscribed lytic lesion (white arrow) in the proximal diaphysis with a narrow zone of transition. It has scalloped margins, suggesting chronicity. No cortical breach is demonstrated. Coronal T2-weighted fat-saturated MR image (B) reveals heterogeneous hyperintense signal of the simple bone cyst (white arrow) with a few thin linear T2-hypointensities (septations; black arrow) within. The bone cyst (white arrow) demonstrates peripheral rim enhancement on the post-contrast T1-weighted fat-saturated image (C).

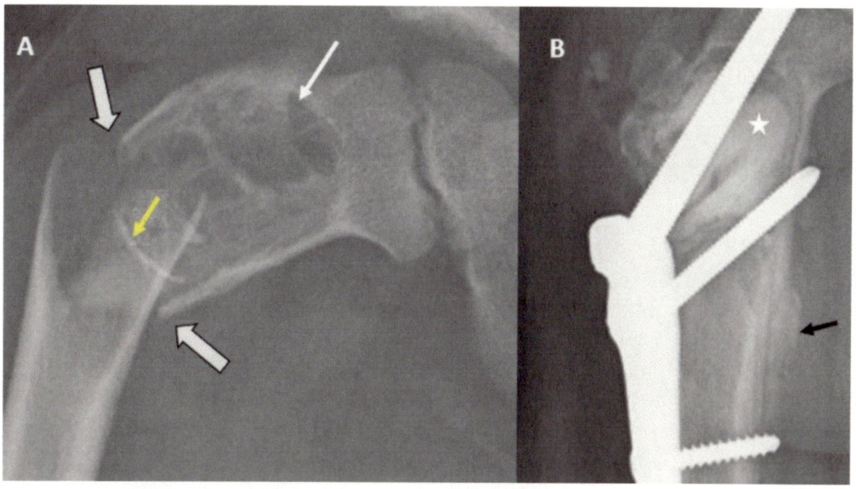

Figure 3.
Simple Bone Cyst: Frontal radiograph of the right femur (A) demonstrates a pathological fracture (thick arrows) through a circumscribed expansile lytic proximal meta-diaphyseal lesion (white arrow). It represents a simple bone cyst with the characteristic fallen-fragment sign (yellow arrow). A follow-up post-treatment frontal radiograph of the right femur (B) shows graft material (white asterisk) cementing the bone cyst and a transfixed healing fracture with good periosteal reaction (black arrow).

The larger cysts with or without fracture are usually treated with curettage and bone grafting [6] (**Figures 1E, 3B**). The fractured cyst tends to heal spontaneously. The prognosis is excellent, although 25% of bone cysts recur after curettage [7]. Cyst aspiration with corticosteroid injection or sclerotherapy has also been used for treatment. Intervention is usually not required for an asymptomatic lesion.

2. Aneurysmal bone cyst:

An aneurysmal bone cyst is a benign, radiolucent, expansile, and hemorrhagic lesion of uncertain etiology. Pathologically, the lesion comprises numerous blood-filled nonendothelialized channels separated by connective tissue of bone or osteoid tissue and osteoclastic giant cells. Aneurysmal bone cyst affects 0.14 per 1,00,000 of the population [8]. There may be a slight female predominance. 75–90% of cases occurred before the age of 20 [9]. The patient usually presents with nonspecific pain and swelling, and a minority of patients (approximately 10%) present with pathological fractures. The lesions are most commonly located in the metaphysis of long bones, the craniofacial bones, and the spine; spinal lesions occur in the posterior elements.

The aneurysmal bone cysts are sharply defined on radiographs and appear as expansile osteolytic lesions with thin sclerotic margins, frequently termed a soap bubble lesion [10] (**Figures 4A, 5A**). If the lesion is wider than the affected normal bone, an ABC should be considered. ABCs are typically multiloculated, and the cortex is usually intact but maybe markedly thinned to the point of being invisible, and the periosteal new bone may be present. CT scan demonstrates these findings better and accurately assesses cortical breach and extension to the soft tissues (**Figure 5C**). Additionally, the CT and MRI demonstrate fluid–fluid levels, which are characteristic of the lesion (**Figures 4C, 5B**). Fluid–fluid levels are due to the dependent location of degraded blood products, especially methemoglobin, which has a much shorter T1 relaxation time than hemoglobin. Fluid–fluid levels may be single

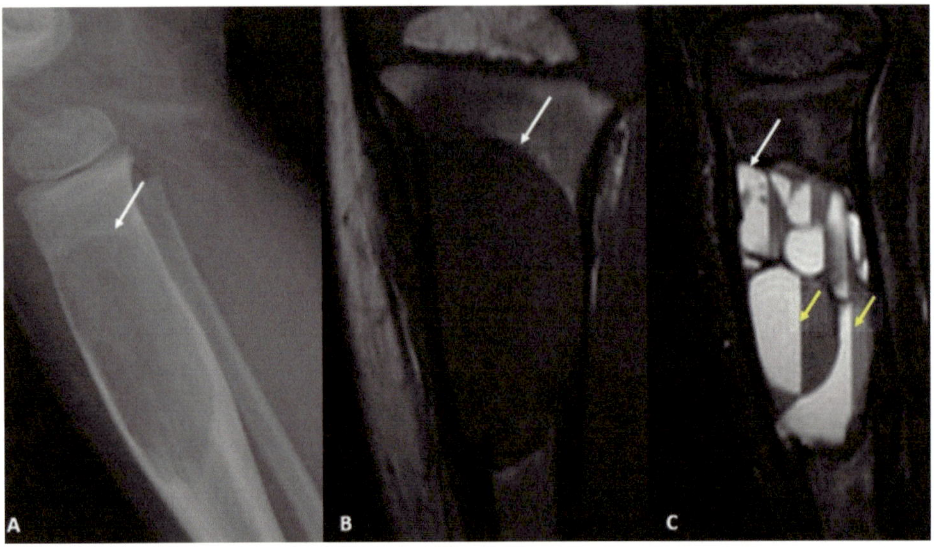

Figure 4.
Aneurysmal Bone Cyst: Lateral radiograph of the left tibia (A) shows a well-circumscribed, expansile, lytic lesion (white arrow) involving the proximal tibial metadiaphysis. It demonstrates internal heterogeneity and has a narrow zone of transition. Coronal T1-weighted image (B) reveals the multiloculated appearance of the lesion (white arrow) and a predominantly intermediate T1 signal. No associated soft tissue swelling is noted. Sagittal fat-saturated T2-weighted image (C) shows multiple fluid-fluid levels within the lesion (yellow arrows), a characteristic imaging feature of an aneurysmal bone cyst.

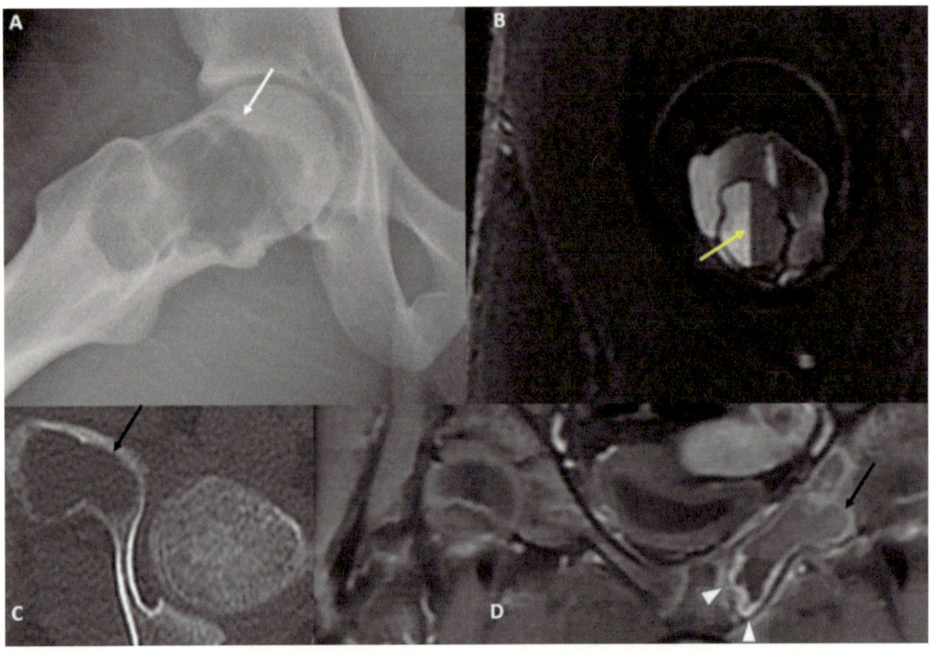

Figure 5.
Aneurysmal Bone Cyst: Lateral radiograph of the pelvis (A) shows an expansile, circumscribed, lytic, proximal femoral metaphyseal lesion (white arrow) with scalloped margins. On axial fat-saturated T2-weighted imaging (B), the lesion shows multiple fluid-fluid levels within (yellow arrow), suggesting an aneurysmal bone cyst. C and D are images of an aneurysmal bone cyst in the left pubic bone in a different patient. The aneurysmal bone cyst appears as a well-circumscribed lytic lesion on CT (C). Coronal T1-weighted fat-saturated post-contrast image (D) depicts heterogeneous and peripheral enhancement of the aneurysmal bone cyst.

or multiple and may be seen as varying horizontal levels within the separate loculations [11]. The signal characteristics of the cyst contents depend on the relative age and concentration of blood components. Abundant hemosiderin may produce areas of low signal. On T1, the cyst is predominantly hypointense (**Figure 4B**). Cyst contents do not enhance, but the septations and wall do (**Figure 5D**).

It may not be possible to differentiate primary and secondary ABCs. Approximately 30% ABC's are secondary [12]. According to one study, the most common reasons for secondary ABC are chondroblastoma and giant cell tumor [13]. Secondary ABC can also be found in other lesions such as osteoblastoma, chondromyxoid fibroma, fibrous dysplasia, and nonossifying fibroma.

Treatment: Most ABCs are treated with curettage and bone grafting. Recurrence rate is approximately 12–30% after initial treatment [14]. Percutaneous treatment with fibrosing agents has also been performed, either in isolation or as a precursor to surgical excision. According to one institution's experience, many ABCs can be treated with polidocanol sclerotherapy [15]. Vascular embolization has also been used. MRI is helpful to identify any solid components which can guide the surgeon for biopsy.

Bone lesions containing osteoid matrix:

1. Enostosis:

Enostosis, also known as the bone island, is a benign focus of compact (cortical) bone located within the cancellous bone (medullary cavity). The bone island is most commonly found incidentally. Pathologically, a bone island is a normal cortical bone containing Haversian canals. There are radiations of cortical bone blending into the normal cancellous bone at the periphery of the lesion. The bone island is likely developmental, a normal cortical bone that fails to resolve during the growth process of endochondral ossification. The bone island is seen in adults far more frequently than children. There is no gender predilection. The bone island is generally a radiographic diagnosis. The bone island is a homogeneously dense lesion on radiography, fading at the periphery and merging into normal marrow. The periphery of the bone island is described as brush-like; may appear somewhat stellate [16] (**Figure 6A**). There is no associated cortical destruction. Polyostotic bone islands concentrated in the metaphyseal region are termed

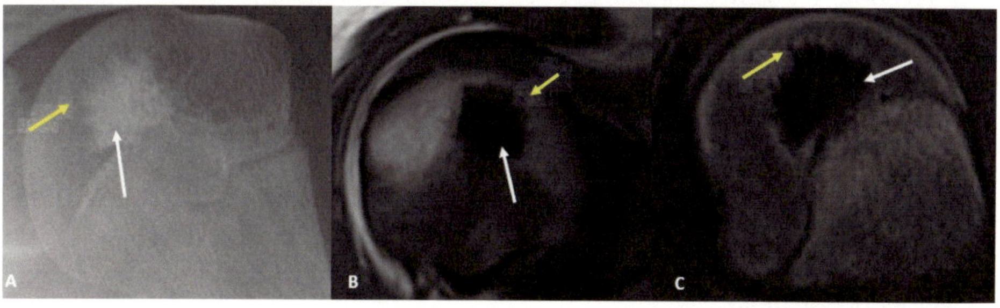

Figure 6.
Enostosis: Frontal radiograph of left humerus (A) shows a circumscribed focal sclerosis (white arrow) in the proximal epiphysis with peripheral brush border extensions into the normal adjacent bone. Axial T1-weighted (B) and T2-weighted fat-saturated (C) images reveal marked hypointense signal of the bone island.

osteopoikilosis. Multiple sclerotic bone lesions can also be seen in patients with tuberous sclerosis complex [17].

On CT scan, enostosis is a sclerotic lesion with peripheral brush border extensions into the normal adjacent bone. Enostosis generally has a mean CT attenuation above 885 Hounsfield units (HU), whereas untreated osteoblastic metastases have mean CT attenuation below 885 HU, according to one study [18]. On MRI, the enostosis demonstrates low signal on all sequences with characteristic peripheral brush border extension into the normal bone (**Figure 6B** and **C**). There is no postcontrast enhancement. On nuclear medicine scintigraphy, if the lesion size is more than 1 cm, increased radiotracer uptake is related to the osteoblastic activity. SPECT CT has a sensitivity of up to 90% in detecting sclerotic bone metastases [19]. No treatment is required for enostosis.

2. Osteoma:

Osteoma is a benign tumor that demonstrates well-differentiated bone formation without aggressive features. Synonyms of osteoma include surface osteoma, parosteal osteoma, ivory osteoma, Ivory exostosis, and hamartoma of bone. Pathologically, osteoma is a hard white dense cortical bone. Many osteomas demonstrate a mixture of bone types. Osteomas may contain cancellous (trabecular, spongy) regions with a thin trabecular architecture with fatty marrow; woven bone with a fairly mature matrix with prominent collagen fibers; and lamellar (compact regions), which have narrow parallel layers of mature bone matrix. Most commonly, osteomas are found incidentally, with less than 5% of osteomas are symptomatic. The symptoms may be related to the mass effect upon the adjacent soft tissue structures, including proptosis, diplopia, sinusitis, mucocele, abscess as a complication of sinus blockage. Osteoma affects all age groups, including children, although most commonly diagnosed in the fourth and fifth decades of life [20]. The male to female ratio is 2:1. More than 75% of osteomas are seen in paranasal sinuses. The most common paranasal sinus affected is the frontal sinus (80% cases) [21]. Gardner syndrome has a known association with osteoma. Gardner syndrome is an autosomal dominant condition in which the patient may also have multiple cutaneous and subcutaneous lesions (cyst, fibromas), desmoid tumors, and multiple colonic polyps (colonic polyps in Gardner's syndrome have a marked propensity to develop adenocarcinoma).

In radiography and CT scan, the osteoma is seen as a homogeneous bone density lesion due to well-differentiated lamellar bone formation. The borders of osteomas are sharply demarcated (**Figure 7A–D**). There is no periosteal reaction. On MRI, osteomas are seen as low signal intensity on all sequences, without enhancement. Enhanced MRI or CT scan is best to evaluate complications such as mucocele, pneumatocele, or abscess. Treatment is required if intracranial or intraorbital extension, location near frontal sinus ostium, more than 50% of the frontal sinus filled by osteoma or unrelenting symptoms [22]. The endoscopic approach for resection is effective in low-grade osteomas. In particular, the open approach, the osteoplastic flap approach, is well tolerated for resection of higher grade osteomas [23].

3. Osteoid Osteoma:

Osteoid osteoma is a benign tumor of osteoblastic origin. The osteoid osteoma is often called "nidus" to distinguish it from surrounding reactive sclerosis from host response. There may be a genetic basis in chromosome band 22q13

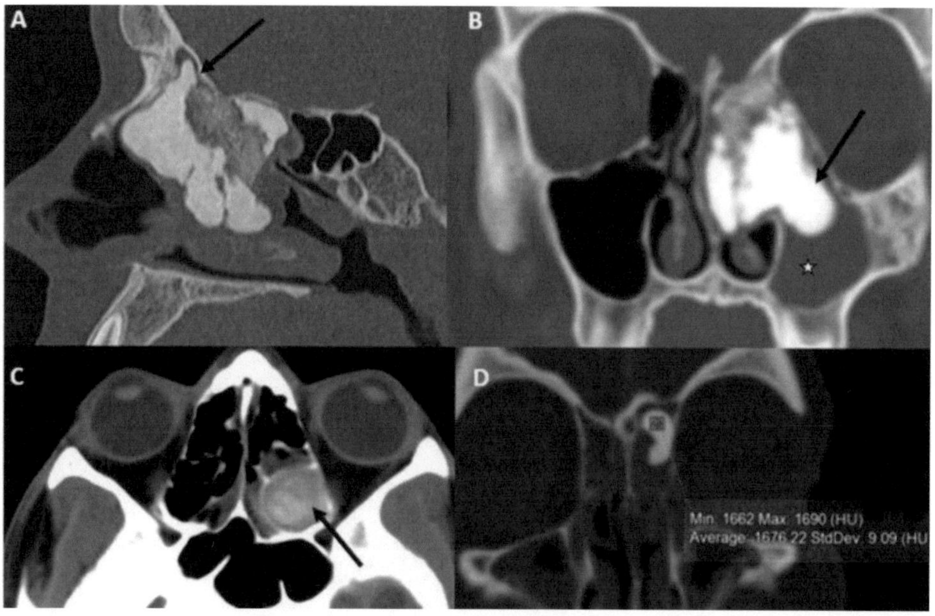

Figure 7.
Osteoma: Sagittal image (bone algorithm, A) and coronal image (bone window, B) of the paranasal sinuses reveal a compact and trabecular sclerotic polypoidal osteoma (black arrows) in the left ethmoid and sphenoid sinuses, extending into the left maxillary sinus with associated occlusion of left osteomeatal unit and left maxillary sinusitis (asterisk). Osteoma can also present as a less dense mass, as depicted by the rounded heterogeneous dense mass in the left posterior ethmoid sinus on the axial CT image (C). Note the high Hounsfield unit of the osteoma (D).

in the patients with osteoid osteoma [24]. The osteoid osteoma contains a central region of vascularized connective tissue that contains osteoblasts and microtrabecular arrays lined by plump appositional osteoblasts. Around the central region, there is a hypervascular sclerotic bone and an abrupt interface between the central lesion and surrounding sclerosis. Osteoid osteoma is relatively common, comprising 5% of all bone tumors and 11% of all benign bone tumors [25]. The most common age range is 10–25 years with a male predilection (Male: female is 3:1) [26]. The classic clinical presentation includes pain, which worsens at night and is relieved by nonsteroidal anti-inflammatory drugs. There is a gradual worsening of the pain over time. Intracapsular lesions may present with signs of synovitis, joint pain, and decreased range of motion. The spinal osteoid osteoma may present with painful nonrotatory scoliosis and concave to the lesion's side [27]. The most common location is cortical diaphyseal, in 65–70% of cases. The most common site involved is femur and tibia, which collectively account for 60% of osteoid osteomas [28]. The nidus is generally less than 2 cm in size.

On radiography, osteoid osteoma appears as an oval lytic lesion located within the dense cortical bone surrounding thickened sclerotic cortical bone (**Figure 8A** and **B**). CT scan helps diagnose and specify the lesion's location (whether cortical versus subperiosteal or medullary) (**Figure 8C** and **D**). CT scan is also helpful to guide percutaneous radiofrequency ablation or cryoablation. The nidus is a round lesion on MRI, slightly hyperintense to muscle on T1-weighted images and hyperintense on T2-weighted images. There is avid arterial phase enhancement of the nidus following contrast administration (**Figure 8E**). The surrounding cortical thickening and reaction is low signal intensity on all sequences. In nuclear medicine scintigraphy, the

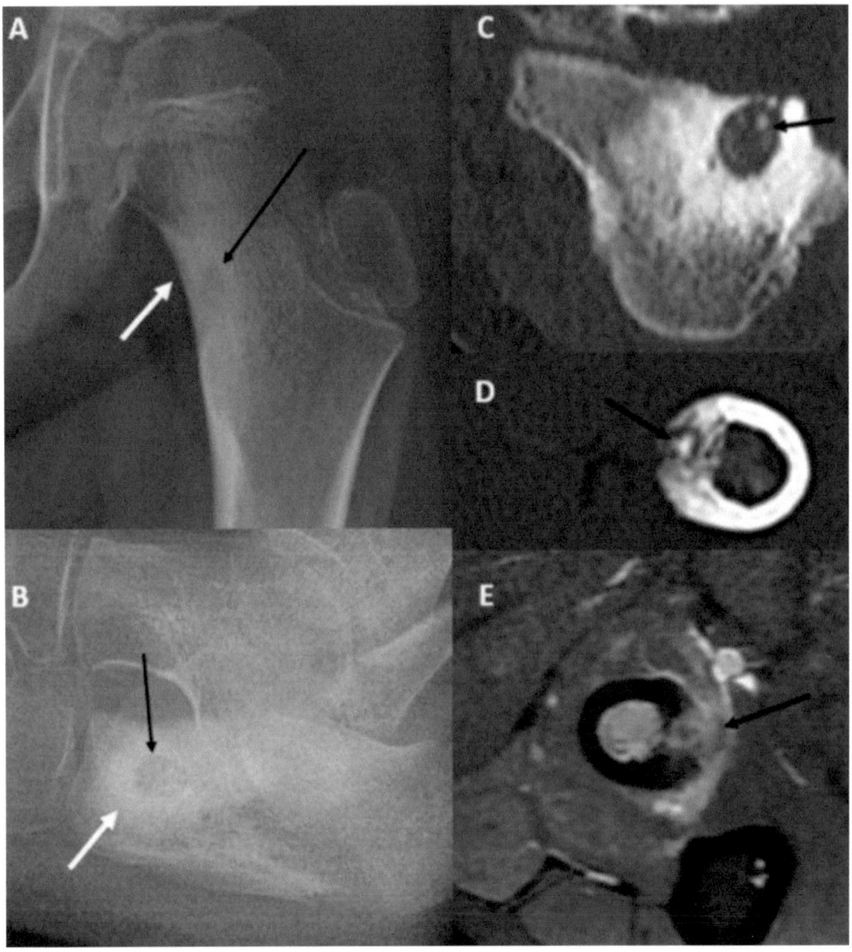

Figure 8.
Osteoid Osteoma: Frontal radiograph of the right femur (A) demonstrates an eccentric lucent area along the medial femoral neck cortex (black arrow) with marginal sclerosis (white arrow). Lateral radiographic view of the calcaneus (B) showing similar lesion with a central lucency surrounded by extensive sclerosis. Axial CT image on the same patient confirms the eccentric location of the lucency that shows an eccentric hyperdense focal speck within, suggesting nidus (C). Osteoid osteoma of the fibula in a different patient appears as a cortical-based lucency with nidus within (black arrow) on axial CT image (D). Axial post-contrast T1-weighted fat-saturated image (E) of the leg at the same level demonstrates enhancement of nidus (black arrow) and adjacent soft tissue.

osteoid osteoma demonstrates intense round activity at the nidus, surrounded by less intensity of reactive bone, often termed as double density sign [29]. The round focus can help distinguish from a stress reaction, which has more linear activity. CT-guided radiofrequency ablation is most likely used to treat osteoid osteomas with an 85–90% initial success rate [30]. Larger or nonspherical lesions may require a second ablative procedure. The CT-guided ablation requires careful planning of an approach to avoid complications. Other alternatives include MR-guided laser ablation or ultrasound ablation.

4. Osteoblastoma:

Osteoblastoma is a rare benign bone-forming tumor, also known as giant osteoid osteoma. Pathologically, osteoblastoma contains elements of osteoid production in the form of active formation of osteoid and immature bone trabeculae. Aggressive osteoblastoma is characterized by epithelioid osteoblasts, which are significantly larger than normal osteoblasts. Histologic differentiation between osteoblastoma and osteoid osteoma may be difficult. The most commonly affected age group is 1st through third decades, with the second decade being the most common [31]. Male:Female ratio is 2.5:1 [32]. The most common presenting symptom is dull, localized, gradually increasing pain. The patient may present with neurologic symptoms if cord or nerve root compression is reported in approximately 50% of spinal lesions [33]. Approximately 30–40% of osteoblastoma occurs in the spine or flat bones [34]. In the spine, posterior elements are most frequently affected (in 94% of cases). The osteoblastoma is usually expanded on imaging, maybe bubbly with a thin cortex and variable degrees of mineralized matrix. There may be a sclerotic margin in the majority of the cases. Matrix ossification and thin cortical rim are more apparent on CT scan than x-ray (**Figure 9A–C**).

On MRI, osteoblastoma is homogeneous low to intermediate signal on T1-weighted images and heterogeneous on fluid sensitive sequences depending on the degree of matrix ossification (**Figure 9D** and **E**). The enhancement ranges from mild to intense depending on the amount of matrix ossification. There may be associated extensive peripheral marrow edema and associated soft tissue edema due to the flare phenomenon [35] (**Figure 10A–C**). On nuclear medicine scintigraphy, osteoblastoma demonstrates intense focal

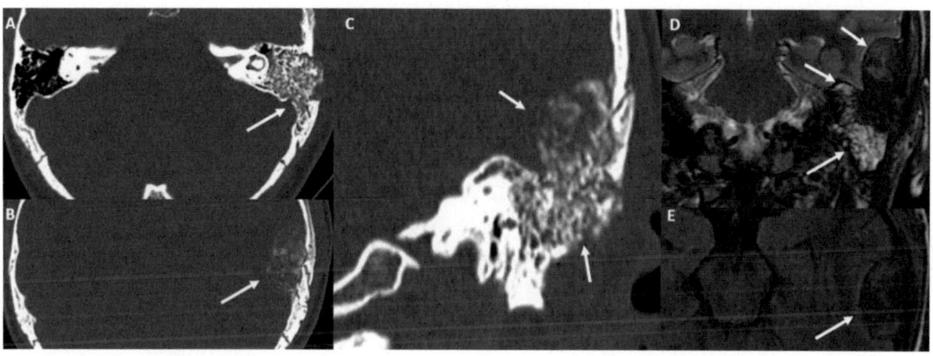

Figure 9.
Osteoblastoma: CT Head axial (A, B) and coronal (C) images in the bone window reveal a circumscribed, expansile, heterogeneous mixed lytic and sclerotic lesion (white arrows) involving the mastoid part of the left temporal bone and has an extradural intracranial component superiorly. Coronal T2-weighted image (D) of the brain at the level of mass (white arrows) reveals heterogenous increased T2 signal of the well-circumscribed mass. Osteoblastoma (white arrow) shows an iso-to-hypointense T1 signal (E).

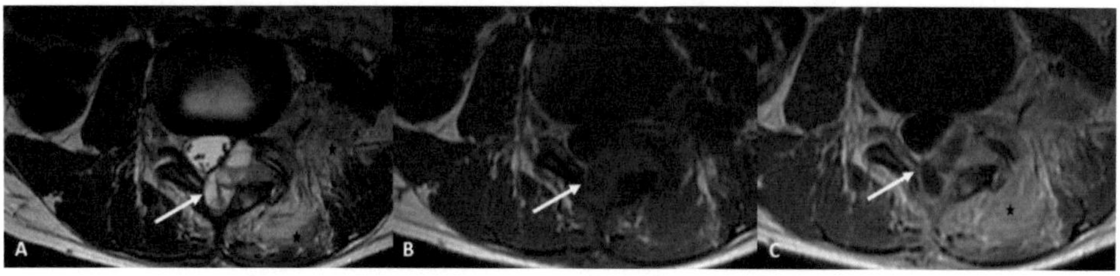

Figure 10.
Osteoblastoma: Axial MR images of the lumbar spine shows an expansile mass lesion involving the left lamina and pedicle, encroaching in the spinal canal. It demonstrates heterogeneous hyperintense T2 signal (white arrow) with subtle fluid-fluid levels (A). The lesion shows an intermediate T1 signal (B) and shows heterogeneous enhancement as depicted in the T1-weighted post-contrast (C). The left posterior paraspinal muscles demonstrate hyperintense T2 signal and post-contrast enhancement (black asterisks).

uptake. Surgical excision, in particular, marginal excision (curettage), is most recommended if wide resection would results in functional impairment. Incomplete excision may result in recurrence (14–24% reported in different series) [36, 37]. Other treatment options include percutaneous thermal ablation. Sporadic cases of osteoblastoma degenerating to osteosarcoma have been reported [38].

Cartilage forming tumors:

1. **Enchondroma:** Enchondroma is a benign tumor of hyaline cartilage originating in the medullary bone. Enchondromas arise from growth plate cartilage rests and/or chondrocytes that subsequently proliferate and slowly enlarge and are composed of mature hyaline cartilage. The most common location of enchondroma is the medullary cavity of tubular bones. Enchondroma accounts for 12–24% of all benign bone tumors and 3–10% of all bone tumors [39, 40]. Approximately 35% of enchondromas occur in hands [40]. In long bones, the proximal humerus is the most common location. Enchondromas are usually detected incidentally on x-ray or MRI. The majority of enchondromas are detected in the third through fifth decades of life [41]. There is no gender predilection. Enchondroma is the most common tumor of the phalanges of the hand. The classic radiographic appearance of enchondroma in the long bones is a metaphyseal lesion with ring and arc type of chondroid mineralization without endosteal scalloping, cortical destruction, or soft tissue mass (**Figure 11A** and **B**). In phalanges, the enchondroma demonstrates an expansile lucent lesion with cortical thinning (**Figure 11D** and **E**). The phalangeal enchondroma may present with pathologic fracture. On MRI, the enchondroma demonstrates low to intermediate signal intensity on T1-weighted images and lobulated high signal on fluid sensitive sequences. Dynamic contrast-enhanced MRI may improve chances of differentiating enchondroma from low-grade chondrosarcoma [42]. Treatment is usually not required for small incidental lesions. For large symptomatic lesions, marginal and/or wide resection should be considered. Sarcoma follow-up surveillance is required if histologic findings showed low-grade chondrosarcoma.

   Ollier disease is a nonhereditary, sporadic skeletal disorder characterized by multiple enchondromas principally located in the metaphyseal regions. If there are associated soft tissue hemangiomas, the syndrome is termed Maffucci syndrome [43]. In Ollier disease, the enchondromas demonstrate vertical streaks of lucencies in the columnar configuration, in metaphases of long bones, extending to the epiphysis [43] (**Figure 12B** and **C**). The phalangeal lesions are typically expansile with sharply defined scalloped margins (**Figure 12A**). There is an approximately 25–30% risk of chondrosarcoma in the setting of Ollier disease [44]. Corrective surgery is required if there are complications such as growth impairment, deformity such as leg length discrepancy.

2. **Chondroblastoma:** Chondroblastoma is a benign cartilage tumor arising in the epiphysis of skeletally immature individuals. More than 75% of chondroblastomas occur in long bones [45]. The most common location is epiphysis, with possible extension to metaphasis. Chondroblastoma may have a genetic basis in structural anomalies involving chromosomes 5 and 8 [46]. Macroscopically, there are nodules of relatively mature cartilage surrounded by highly cellular tissue. Giant cells are usually present in the tumor. The most

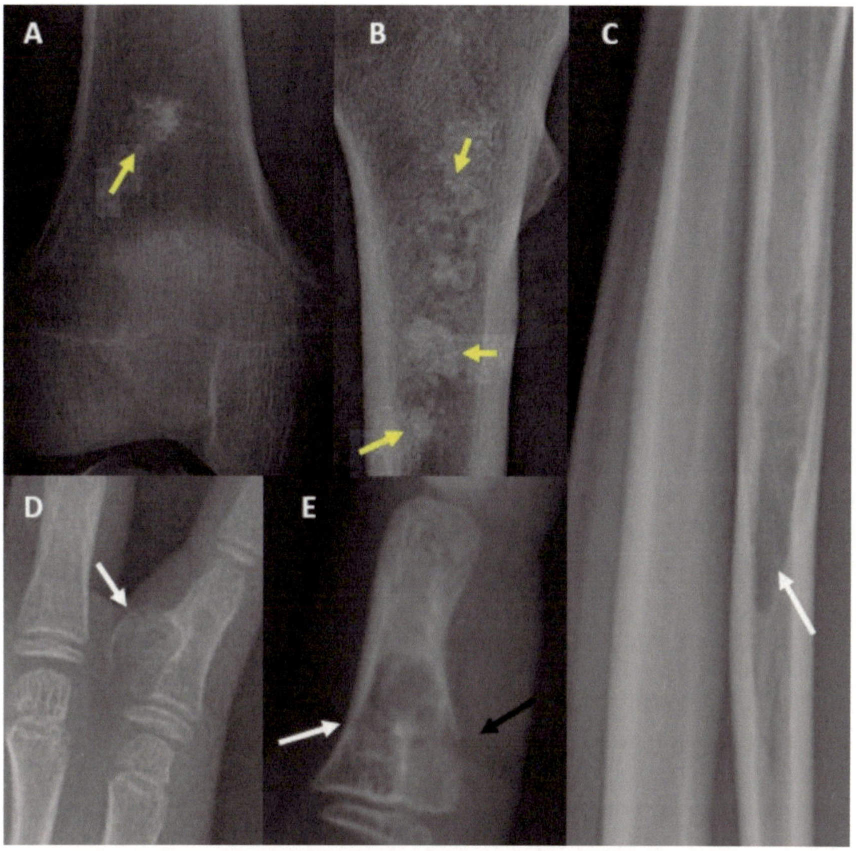

Figure 11.
Enchondroma: Frontal radiograph of the distal femur (A) and proximal femur (B) in two different patients reveal the characteristic rings and arcs pattern of chondroid mineralization (yellow arrows). The lateral radiograph of the forearm (C) shows an expansile lytic lesion (white arrow) in the mid-diaphysis of radius. It demonstrates a narrow zone of transition without any periosteal reaction or associated soft tissue swelling. A frontal radiographic view of the proximal phalanx of the little finger (D) shows a well-defined eccentric osteolytic lesion (white arrow). The frontal radiograph of the index finger (E) shows an expansile well-circumscribed osteolytic lesion (white arrow) with a chondroid matrix. The black arrow points to a cortical breach concerning a pathological fracture.

common presenting symptom is mild localized pain, which refers to joint. The most common age range affected is 10–25 years old. Males are more frequently affected than females (nearly 2:1). Chondroblastoma comprises less than 1% of all bone tumors and approximately 9% of benign bone tumors [47]. The chondroblastoma is a geographic lytic lesion with sclerotic margins in most lesions on radiography and CT scan. The lesion may contain chondroid matrix calcifications. The lesions are eccentrically located within the epiphysis with extension into metadiaphysis as they enlarge. There may be an associated cortical expansion or thinning (**Figure 13A–C**). On MRI, the lesions are typically low signal on T1 and inhomogeneously high signal on fluid sensitive sequences. The inhomogeneity is related to the chondroid matrix, calcification, and fluid within the lesion [48] (**Figure 13D–F**). Curettage and bone grafting is the surgical treatment of choice. Radiofrequency ablation may be considered in small lesions.

3. **Chondromyxoid fibroma:** Chondromyxoid fibroma is a benign lobulated cartilaginous tumor. Approximately 60% of chondromyxoid fibromas occur in long bones, with the proximal tibia being the single most frequent site. Genetic basis has been described in the literature in the form of clonal abnormalities of

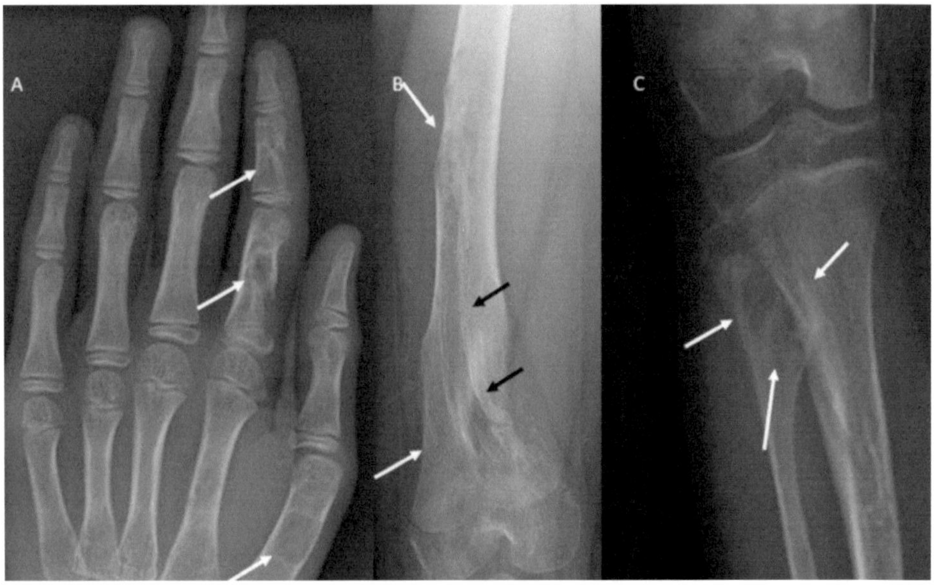

Figure 12.
Ollier's disease: Frontal radiograph of the left hand (A) demonstrates multiple circumscribed lucent areas (white arrows) in hand with a sharp zone of transition. Frontal radiograph of the right femur (B) shows vertical streaks of lucencies (black arrows) extending from diaphysis towards epiphysis. Frontal radiograph of the right tibia and fibula (C) reveals an expansile enchondroma in the proximal fibular metaphysis (white arrows) and a not that much expansile enchondroma in the tibial metadiaphysis.

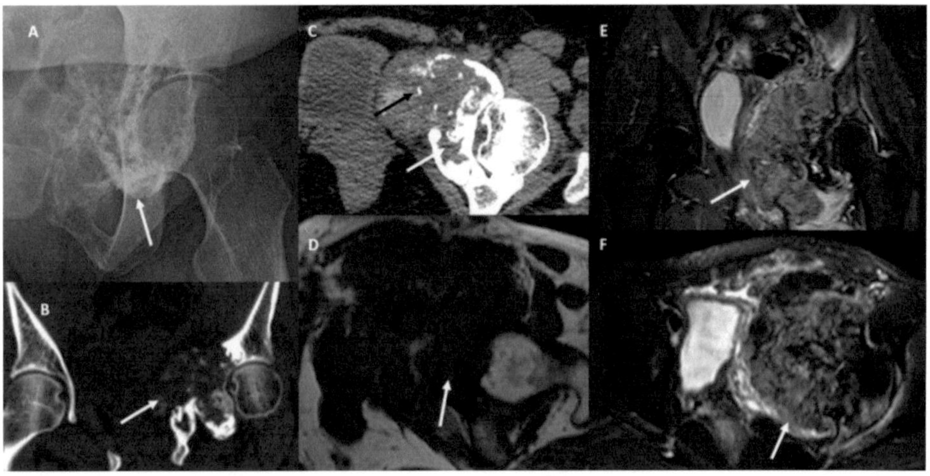

Figure 13.
Chondroblastoma: Frontal radiographic view of the left pelvis (A) shows a calcified mass of the left ischium and pubic bones. Coronal bone window (B) and axial soft tissue window (C) images demonstrate an expansile osteolytic lesion (white arrows) with a well-defined lobulated margin and chondroid matrix (black arrow). Chondroblastoma demonstrates a hypointense T1 signal (white arrow; D) with a peripheral sclerotic rim. Coronal (E) and axial (F) T2-weighted fat-saturated images reveal heterogeneous hyperintense T2 signal of the mass (white arrows) with extensive peritumoral edema.

chromosome 6 and pronounced expression of type II collagen, which is unique compared with other cartilaginous lesions. Microscopically, the lesion is lobular with stellate cells in the myxoid background. The most common presenting symptom is mild chronic pain. The mean age of presentation is 23 years, with 50 percent of patients are in the second decade at presentation. There is slight medial predominance. On radiography and CT, the lesions are

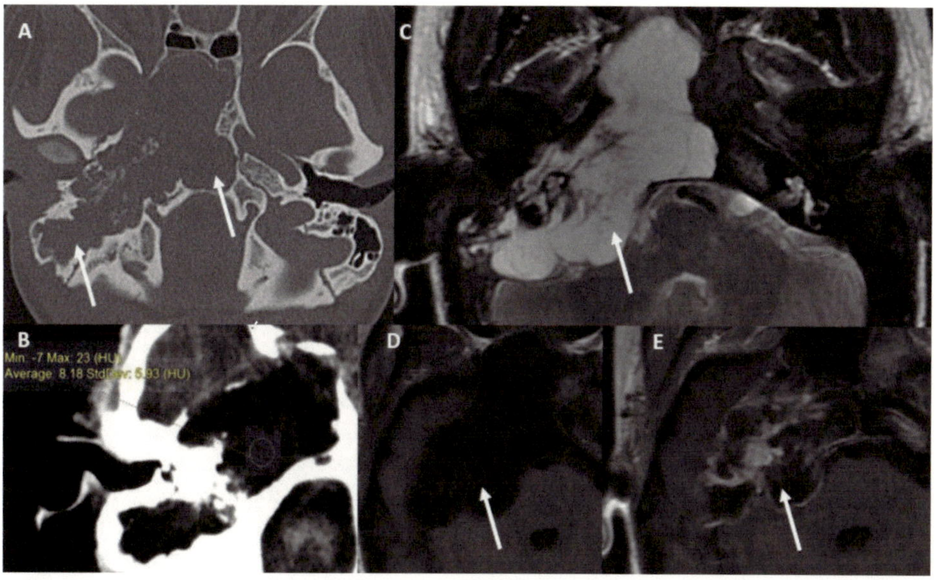

Figure 14.
Chondromyxoid fibroma: Bone window (A) and soft tissue window (B) axial CT head images show a well-defined lobulated lytic lesion (white arrows) involving the mastoid and petrous parts of the right temporal bone and clivus. A note is made of the low attenuation value of the CMF lesion and absent calcifications. On the T2-weighted image (C), the CMF lesion demonstrates a peripheral hypointense sclerotic rim with an intrinsic high signal (white arrow). It shows a hypointense T1 signal (D) and shows thick peripheral enhancement (E). MR features to support the diagnosis of the chondromyxoid fibroma (CMF).

geographic with sclerotic margins. The lesions typically occur in metaphysis or diaphysis, which are oriented along the longitudinal axis of the bone. Approximately 60% of lesions are eccentric, with evidence of lobulation and thinning of the cortex (**Figure 14A** and **B**). Pseudotrabeculations within the lesion give the appearance of septations [49]. There is an absence of periosteal reaction without pathologic fracture. On MRI, the lesion is typically isointense to skeletal muscle on T1-weighted images, and on fluid sensitive sequences, the lesion is centrally hyperintense with a peripheral band of intermediate signal. There is a peripheral nodular enhancement or diffuse postcontrast enhancement [50] (**Figure 14C–E**). The lesions are typically treated with marginal excision with curettage and bone grafting. The recurrence rate is approximately 3–22% [51].

4. **Osteochondroma:** Osteochondroma is cartilage capped exostosis with continuous cortex and marrow extending from the underlying bone. Osteochondroma most commonly arises from metaphysis or metaphyseal equivalents. Approximately 95% of them are located in extremities; the femur is most commonly affected [52]. Microscopically, the inner layer is composed of normal bone; the middle layer is composed of cartilage cap with superficial clusters of chondrocytes, and the outer layer is composed of perichondrium, which is continuous with the periosteum of the underlying bone. The most common presenting symptom is a chronically present hard swelling. It may present as mechanical pain from trauma or impingement. Vascular complications include pseudoaneurysm formation and arterial or venous stenosis/thrombosis. Increasing pain and/or mass enlargement following skeletal maturation suggest degeneration to chondrosarcoma [53]. Osteochondromas could be sessile or pedunculated. On radiography and CT scan, the pedunculated osteochondroma

demonstrates a narrow stalk with cauliflower exostosis (**Figure 15D**), and the sessile osteochondroma is broad-based (**Figure 15A** and **C**). If near the joint, osteochondroma tends to project away from the joint line, growing along the forces generated by the location of the tendons and ligaments. The pelvic osteochondromas could become very large before discovery. Rib lesions may present with pneumothorax. Endochondral calcification may be seen within the cartilage cap and medullary bone as the rings and arcs, punctate or flocculant calcification. The overlying cartilage cap is generally thinned, not evaluated by radiograph. Degeneration of the lesion to chondrosarcoma is suggested by osseous destruction, change in calcifications, or enlargement of the cartilage cap as evidenced by distortion of the fat planes. On MRI, the cortex of the lesion is contiguous with the underlying bone. The overlying hyaline cartilage cap has a lobulated high signal on fluid-sensitive sequences covered by thin perichondrium and demonstrates a low signal on T1 and T2 sequences [54] (**Figure 15E** and **F**). Surgical resection of the osteochondroma is recommended when the cartilage cap thickness is greater than 1 cm. In one study, the use of 2 cm as a cutoff for distinguishing benign osteochondromas from secondary chondrosarcomas provided sensitivities, specificities, positive predictive values, and negative predictive values of 100%, 98%, 96%, and 100%, respectively, for MR imaging and 100%, 95%, 93%, and 100%, respectively, for CT [54]. Treatment is mostly watchful waiting. Resection of the osteochondroma is recommended when there are mechanical complications such as bursa formation, nerve irritation, or impingement. Resection of the entire perichondrium is required to avoid recurrence. Chondrosarcoma is typically treated by wide surgical resection.

Multiple hereditary exostoses, also known as diaphyseal aclasis, is an autosomal dominant condition in which there are multiple sessile and pedunculated osteochondromas. Approximately 90% of patients have a positive family history of this condition [55]. There is a symmetric widening of the metaphysis with the normal underlying bone. Sessile osteochondromas

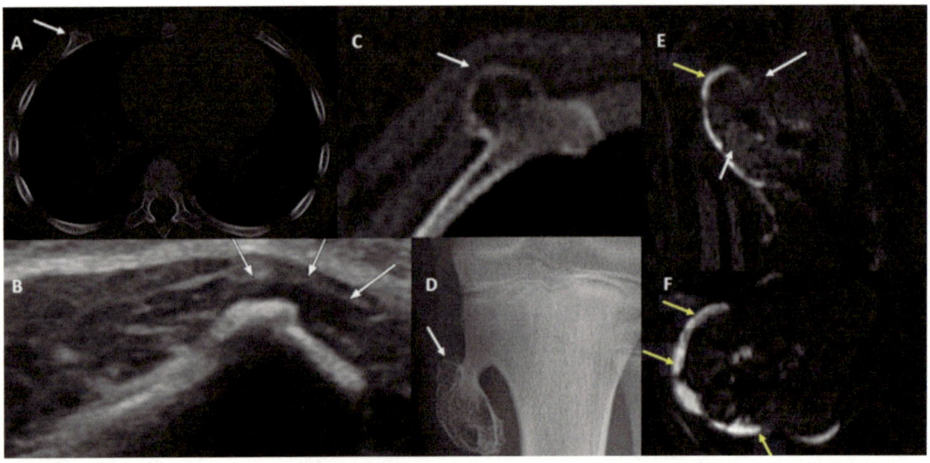

Figure 15.
Osteochondroma: Axial CT bone algorithm image (A) of the mid thorax shows a focal bulge in the anterior right rib (white arrow) with cortical continuity, a finding also appreciated on the longitudinal grayscale ultrasound image (B). It represents a sessile osteochondroma, another example of which is C (white arrow). Frontal radiograph of the left tibia (D) reveals a pedunculated osteochondroma (white arrow) noted in the metaphyseal region, with the cortex of the parent bone (tibia in this case) contiguous with that of the lesion, and the lesion is directed away from the joint. The T2-weighted fat-saturated coronal (E) and axial (F) images reveal the T2 hyperintense cartilage cap (yellow arrows) of that osteochondral lesion (white arrows).

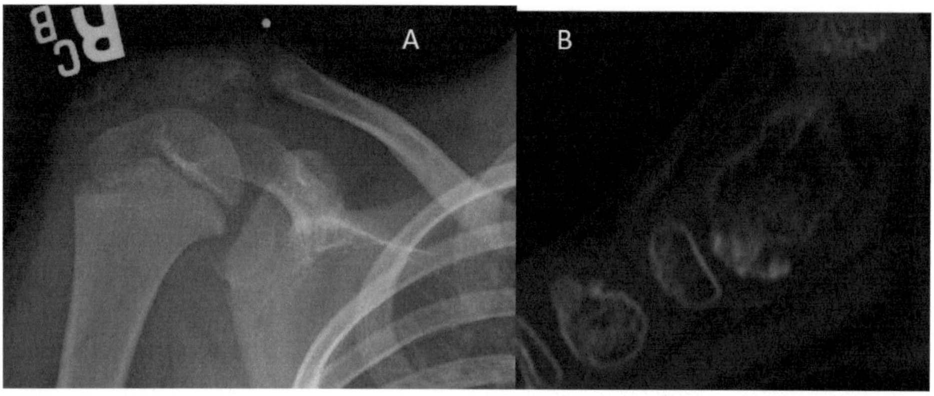

Figure 16.
Trevor disease: Frontal radiograph of the right shoulder demonstrates an osteochondroma arising from right proximal humeral epiphysis, suggesting Trevor Disease (A). Sagittal bone window image of ankle demonstrates an osteochondroma arising from Talus (B).

are more common than pedunculated osteochondromas. There is an approximately 3–5% incidence of degeneration to chondrosarcoma [56]. Radiography is the 1st line modality to evaluate for this condition. MRI can be performed to evaluate the thickness of the cartilage cap and evaluate for complications from the mass effect. If the lesion is superficial, ultrasound can also be used to evaluate for thickness and irregularity of the cartilage cap. Surgical resection is performed if there are complications from mass effect or evidence of degeneration to chondrosarcoma.

Trevor disease, also known as dysplasia epiphysealis hemimelica, is an extremely rare, nonhereditary disease in which the osteochondromas arise from the epiphysis. It affects approximately one in 1 million population [57]. Only one epiphysis is involved in the localized type, although multiple epiphyses are affected involving the entire extremity in generalized type. There is the presence of an exostosis arising from the epiphysis on radiography and CT scan (**Figure 16A** and **B**). Surgical excision of mass is usually performed to preserve the joint.

5. **Juxtacortical chondroma:** Juxtacortical chondroma is a chondroid tumor arising in the periosteal layer of tubular bones. It is a rare benign tumor comprising less than 2% of chondromas [58]. The most common age range affected is second through fourth decades. Although, it may occur in children. Juxtacortical chondroma is a surface lesion arising from the metaphysis of the tubular bone-producing chondroid matrix. The lesion is located in the proximal humerus and femur in 70% of cases. On radiography, there is saucerization of the cortex with sclerotic margins and matrix calcification (in 75% of cases) (**Figure 17A**). There may be associated soft tissue mass. On MRI, the lesion is lobulated with iso to hypointense T1 signal and hyperintense T2 signal with heterogeneous predominantly peripheral enhancement (**Figure 17B–E**). The tumor demonstrates slow local progression. Wide surgical excision is the most appropriate treatment for lesions greater than 3 cm in size [59].

Fibro-osseous lesions:

1. **Fibrous cortical defect:** Fibrous cortical defect is the most common benign bone lesion [60]. The most common location is usually metaphysis or

metadiaphysis junction of the femur or tibia. On radiographs, the fibrous cortical defects are eccentric cortically based lucent lesions with mineralized rim (**Figure 18A** and **B**). There is no involvement of the underlying medullary cavity. There is no periosteal reaction. The fibrous cortical defects are typically hypointense on T1 weighted images and hyperintense on T2-weighted images (**Figure 18C** and **D**). The signal intensity depends on the stage of healing. Fibrous cortical defects are typically seen incidentally on radiographs. These are no-touch lesions (no treatment is required). Benign fibro-osseous lesions may be metabolically active on FDG PET CT exam and should not be confused with metastases [61].

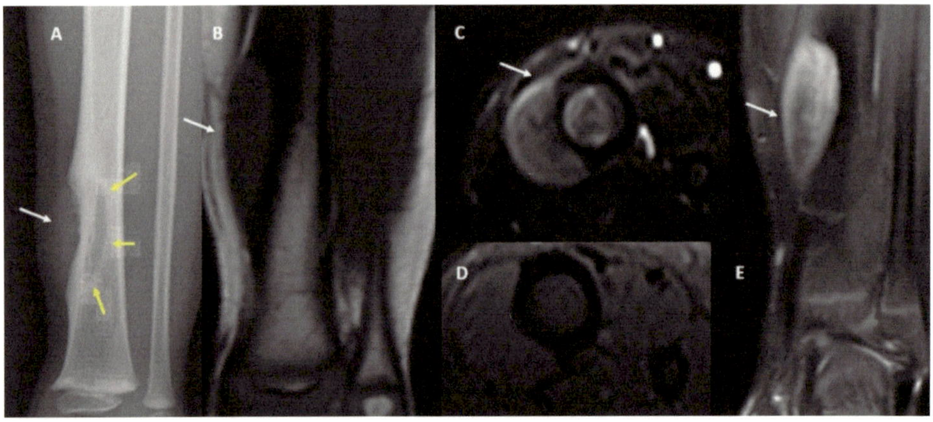

Figure 17.
Juxtacortical chondroma: Frontal radiograph of the left tibia and fibula (A) demonstrates a well-defined distal tibial metadiaphyseal lucent lesion (white arrow) with underlying cortical saucerization or scalloping(yellow arrows) and subjacent cortical sclerosis. It demonstrates a hypointense T1 signal (B) and an increased T2 signal (C). T1-weighted fat-saturated pre (D) and postcontrast (E) images demonstrate peripheral enhancement of the chondroma lesion (white arrow).

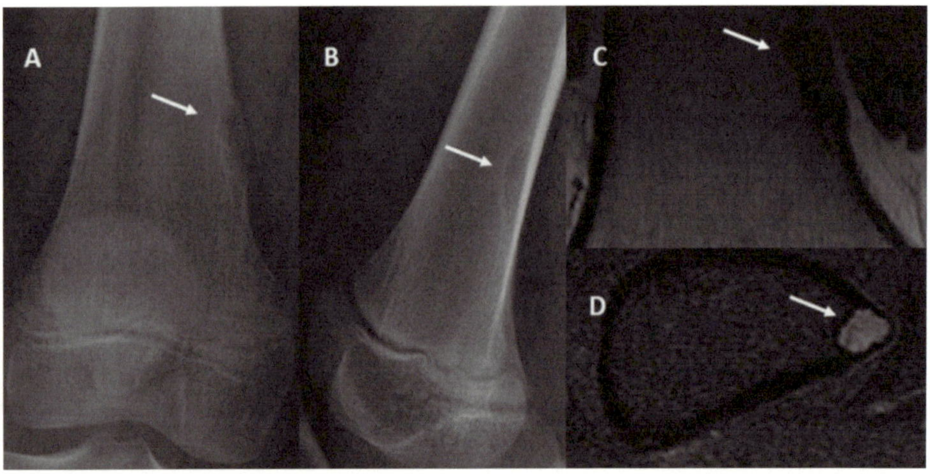

Figure 18.
Fibrous cortical defect: Frontal (A) and lateral (B) radiographs of distal femur demonstrate eccentric lucent intracortical defect (white arrows) outlined by a rim of sclerosis. Note that there is no involvement of the underlying medullary cavity, and there is no periosteal reaction. The lesion (white arrows) demonstrates a hypointense T1 signal (C) and increased T2 signal with a peripheral hypointense sclerotic rim (D).

2. **Nonossifying fibroma:** Nonossifying fibroma is a benign fibrous lesion composed of spindle cells in a collagenous matrix. Nonossifying fibroma is generally greater than 3 cm in greatest dimension (as opposed to a fibrous cortical defect less than 3 cm in diameter) [62]. Nonossifying fibroma typically originates in the metaphysis and is cortically based, most commonly found around the knee and distal tibia. It can be multifocal in 8% of cases. Multifocal nonossifying fibromas may be associated with neurofibromatosis (Jaffe-Campanacci syndrome). Nonossifying fibroma is usually asymptomatic; however, it could present with pathological fracture. It is typically seen in the first and second decade of life.

   Radiographic and CT appearance depends on the morphologic age of the lesion. Initially, the lesion appears as a lytic, geographic area with a thin sclerotic margin (**Figure 19A** and **B**). During early filling phases, it has a thicker sclerotic margin forming peripheral bone. During late stages, the lesion may be entirely sclerotic with usual remodeling to normal bone type appearance. On MRI, the lesion is hypointense to skeletal muscle on T1 and heterogeneous on fluid sensitive sequences with low signal areas and hyperintense areas (**Figure 19C** and **D**). The regions of low signal areas are fibrous elements and hemosiderin. There is peripheral and septal enhancement following contrast administration. No cortical destruction or soft tissue mass lesion is demonstrated. No treatment is required in a vast majority of cases. If there is a risk for pathologic fracture due to the size of the lesion, curettage and bone grafting can be performed. Syndromic form of multiple nonossifying fibromas has a higher rate of recurrence after surgical removal [63].

3. **Fibrous Dysplasia**: Fibrous dysplasia (FD) is a developmental disorder characterized by the replacement of normal bone by immature bone and cartilaginous tissue. Most cases are sporadic and are related to a mutation in the GNAS1 gene. GNAS gene codes for the stimulatory alpha subunit of guanine nucleotide-binding protein, and its mutation result in persistent adenyl cyclase activation leading to osteoblastic proliferation. FD comprises

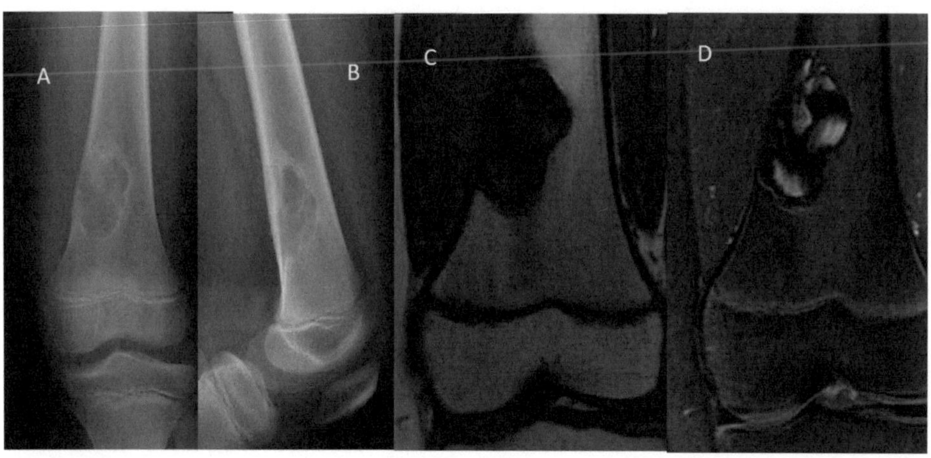

Figure 19.
Non-Ossifying Fibroma: Frontal and lateral radiographs of femur demonstrate an eccentric cortically based radiolucent lesion with sclerotic margin in distal meta-diaphysis (A, B). On MRI of the same patient, the lesion demonstrates predominantly hypointense signal on T1 and heterogenous signal on STIR due to fibrous elements and hemosiderin (C, D).

about 5–7% of all cases of benign tumors [64]. It can involve any bone and any part of the bone.

Four clinical presentations of FD have been described [65]:

1. Monostotic FD (70–80% of all FD): Single bone is involved (**Figure 20**) with craniofacial involvement in 10–27% of cases. It generally manifests at 10–30 years of age. FD lesions do not demonstrate an increase in size after puberty.

2. Polyostotic FD (20–25%): Multiple bones are affected (**Figure 21**). Craniofacial involvement is seen in 40–100% of cases. It usually manifests before age 10. Polyostotic FD lesions, in some cases, increase in size even after puberty.

3. McCune-Albright syndrome (3%): It is characterized by café-au-lait skin macules, polyostotic fibrous dysplasia, and endocrine hyperfunction disorders (precocious puberty, pituitary adenomas secreting growth hormone, hyperthyroidism, and autonomous adrenal hyperplasia). Increased growth and recurrence of the FD lesions are seen [66]. Some examples include the classic "Shepherd's crook" deformity of the femur, coxa vara, and scoliosis resulting from spinal FD.

4. Mazabraud syndrome: It is characterized by the coexistence of polyostotic fibrous dysplasia lesion and intramuscular myxomas.

Generally, FD lesions are lytic and well-defined but can look like almost anything and are not associated with soft tissue swelling. The radiographical features of FD can vary from ground-glass appearance, purely cystic (completely lucent) lesions, mixed cystic and sclerotic lesions, to sclerotic lesions. They may demonstrate a geographic (circumscribed) pattern with or without a sclerotic border or appear as expanded lesions with or without associated endosteal scalloping. CT accurately delineates margins of the FD lesions and helps in detecting subtle fractures [67]. FD lesions demonstrate different CT patterns depending upon the patient's age, varying from homogeneous dense lesions in the pre-pubertal life to a

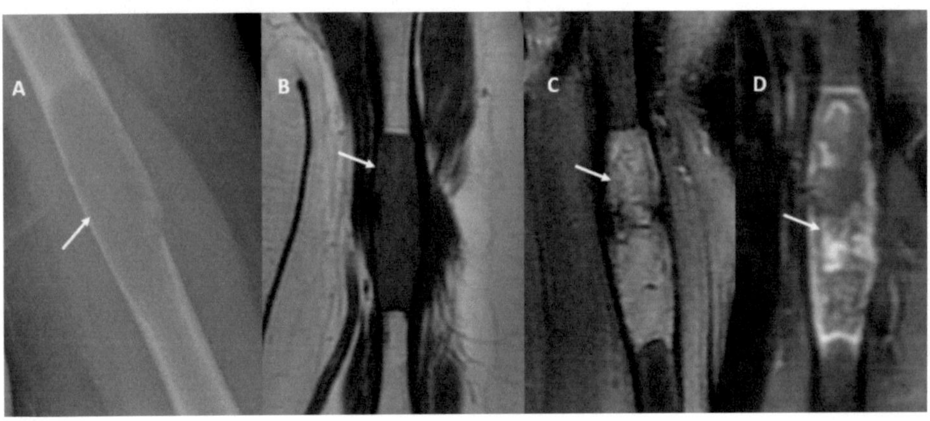

Figure 20.
Fibrous dysplasia: Left humerus radiograph (A) demonstrates an expansile diaphyseal lesion (white arrow) with a ground-glass matrix. The lesion (white arrows) demonstrates hypointense T1 signal (B), heterogeneous but predominantly increased T2 signal (C), and heterogeneous postcontrast enhancement (D).

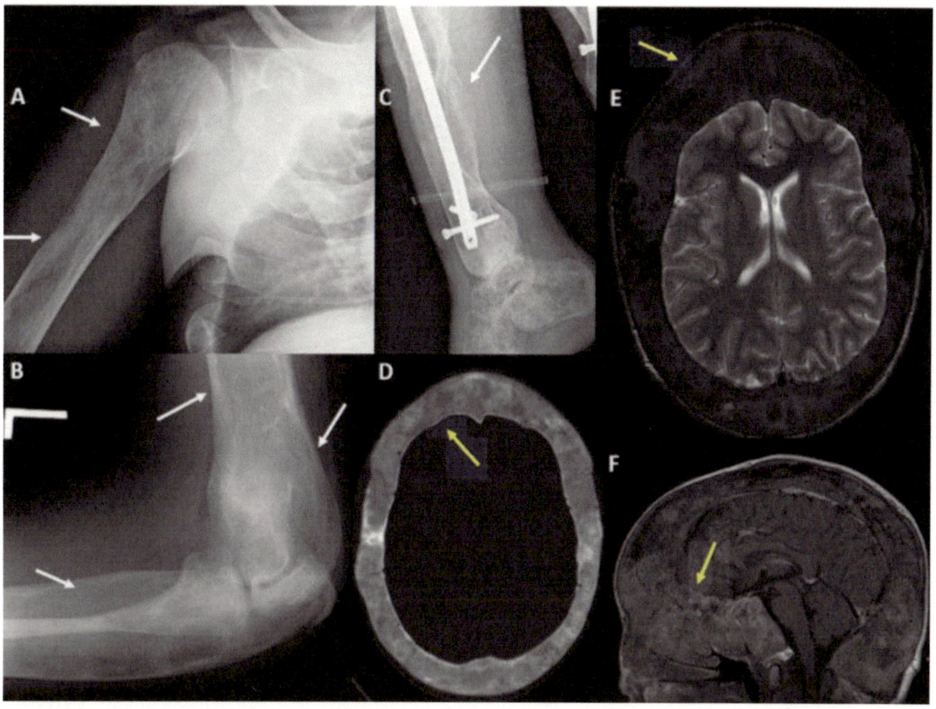

Figure 21.
McCune Albright syndrome: Radiographs (A–C) of the right humerus, left elbow and distal leg demonstrate extensive polyostotic fibrous dysplasia (white arrows) with associated deformities. Axial CT head bone algorithm image (D) demonstrates the characteristic ground-glass appearance of the cranium (yellow arrow) and diffuse widening of diploic space. Axial T2-weighted MR image (E) reveals a heterogenous mixed pattern of low and high SI within the expansile lesion. Also demonstrated is the heterogeneous T1 signal of the thickened calvarium (yellow arrow) in fibrous dysplasia (F).

mixed lucent-dense pattern between ages of 10–20 years, and some of these lesions may appear ground-glass in adult life. Diagnosing FD lesions purely by MRI is highly challenging because of the highly variable signal demonstrated by these lesions. Typically, the T1 signal is related to the ratio of fibrous tissue to the mineralized matrix, with the FD lesions with high fibrous component showing an intermediate T1 signal, compared to the low signal intensity of lesions with the highly mineralized matrix. The metabolically active fibrous component appears hyperintense on T2-weighted imaging and demonstrates intense enhancement because of high vascularity [68]. Franz et al. described the "milk cloud appearance" of the ground-glass FD lesions on contrast-enhanced T1-weighted MR imaging [69].

Active FD lesions demonstrate increased uptake on 18F-FDG PET/CT imaging (18F-NaF is a bone-seeking positron-emitting radiopharmaceutical) which is currently the imaging modality of choice to evaluate FD activity [70].

In most cases, no treatment is required. Curettage and bone grafting is an option if there is a risk for pathologic fracture due to the size of the FD lesion. Persistent moderate-to-severe bone pain of FD can be controlled by intravenous bisphosphonate therapy. However, it should be started only after ensuring the normocalcemic status of the patient and dental evaluation (to decrease the risk of osteonecrosis of the jaw) [71].

3.1 Histiocytic/Langerhans cell lesions

Langerhans cell histiocytosis (LCH)/Eosinophilic granuloma: Langerhans cell histiocytosis is neoplastic proliferation of Langerhans cells/histiocytes in the

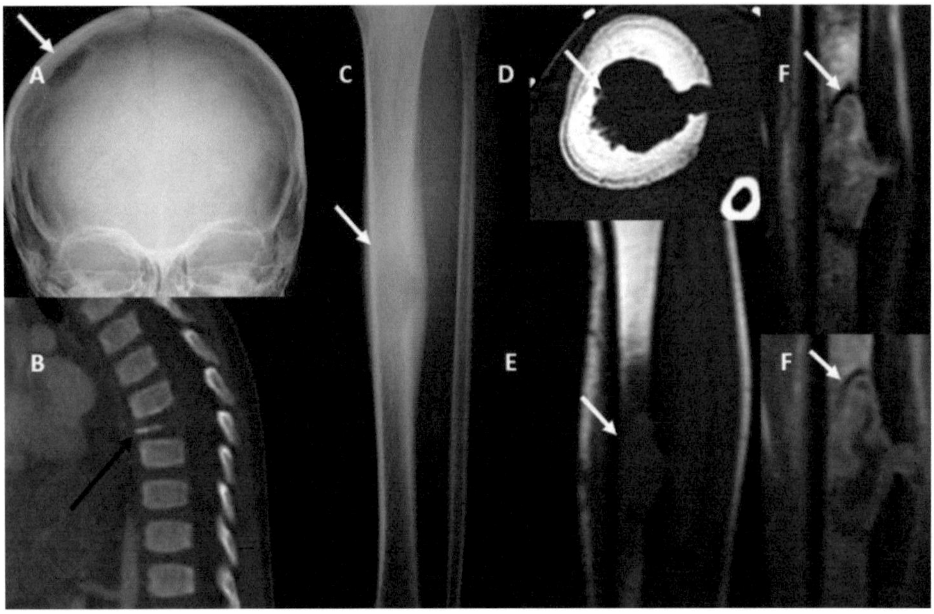

Figure 22.
Eosinophilic granuloma: Skull radiograph (A) demonstrates a punched-out lucent lesion (white arrow) without a mineralized rim. Sagittal bone window image of the thoracic spine (B) reveals a collapsed vertebral body, namely "vertebra plana" (black arrow). Frontal radiograph of left tibia (C) showing an expansile well-defined osteolytic diaphyseal lesion (white arrow)with a benign periosteal reaction. Axial CT bone window image (D) at the level of the diaphyseal lesion demonstrates a punched-out lucent lesion (white arrow). MR images reveal intermediate T1 signal (E), heterogeneous increased T2 signal (F), and thick peripheral enhancement (F).

reticuloendothelial system. These cells produce prostaglandins which are responsible for medullary bone resorption. The incidence of LCH is approximately 1 in 200 000 children [72]. Flat bones are most commonly involved in approximately 65–70% of cases. Skull is the most common site of involvement in flat bones. The monostotic form is more common, seen in approximately 70% of cases [73]. The mean age at diagnosis is typically 5–10 years. Classic radiographic/CT appearance includes solitary or multiple punched-out skull lesions without sclerotic rim (**Figure 22A**). There is a typical beveled edge appearance due to the asymmetrical involvement of inner and outer tables. Spinal lesions may present with vertebra plana (complete collapse and flattening of vertebral body) (**Figure 22B**). When present in long bones, the eosinophilic granuloma is a permeative aggressive appearing lesion with possible associated endosteal scalloping, periosteal reaction, and soft tissue mass (**Figure 22C** and **D**). The lesion may present in any part of bone but most commonly affects diaphysis. On MRI, these lesions are hypointense on T1, hyperintense on T2/STIR with diffuse post-contrast enhancement (**Figure 22E–G**). Whole-body PET/CT can be utilized to evaluate polyostotic disease and monitor for response to therapy. LCH commonly undergoes spontaneous resolution. If the symptoms persist, excision and curettage are the treatment of choice.

3.2 Giant cell lesions

Giant cell tumor: Giant cell tumor (GCT) of bone, a benign but locally aggressive tumor, comprises multinucleated giant cells interspersed with mononuclear stromal cells. It comprises 20% of all benign bone tumors and 5% of all primary bone tumors. GCT is more prevalent in females and between 20 and 30 years (80%

of cases occur between 20 and 50 years of age). It is rarely seen in the pediatric age group (3% of cases occur before age 14). Though GCT mainly involves long bones, any bone can be affected. The most common location of GCT is around the knee (distal femur and proximal tibia), followed by the distal radius and sacrum [74].

Campanacci and Enneking's clinic radiological staging of GCT: Stage I-The lesion is restricted to the marrow, and bone contour is not affected (cortex may be thinned out); Stage II- Cortical bulging without any signs of rupture; Stage III- Cortical breach with an invasion of soft tissues [75].

Typical radiographic presentation of GCT is that of a circumscribed, eccentric, epiphyseal lytic lesion that extends to the subchondral bone in patients with closed physis. GCT demonstrates a "soap bubble" appearance on radiographs and CT because of bony septae (**Figure 23A** and **B**). The MR features of GCT are nonspecific. Most commonly, GCT shows hypointense T1 signal and heterogeneous T2 signal (due to collagen content of fibrous components of GCT and deposition of hemosiderin) [76] (**Figure 23C–F**). Contrast administration helps in delineating solid and cystic components. On scintigraphy, there is increased Technetium 99 m–methylene diphosphonate uptake along the periphery of the lesion with central photopenia. An aggressive GCT may demonstrate expansile remodeling, cortical thinning or destruction, a wide zone of transition, and associated soft tissue. Fluid–fluid levels within GCT suggest secondary aneurysmal bone cyst (ABC) formation.

Though intralesional procedures (such as curettage and cement placement) are a preferred approach to treat GCT, they are complicated by recurrence because of residual tumor tissue. He et al. described marginal infiltration as the "paintbrush borders" sign on MRI and advocated it as an independent prognostic factor for local recurrence of GCTB after intralesional curettage [77]. In advanced GCT, Denosumab is recommended for immediate local control and facilitates surgery later [78].

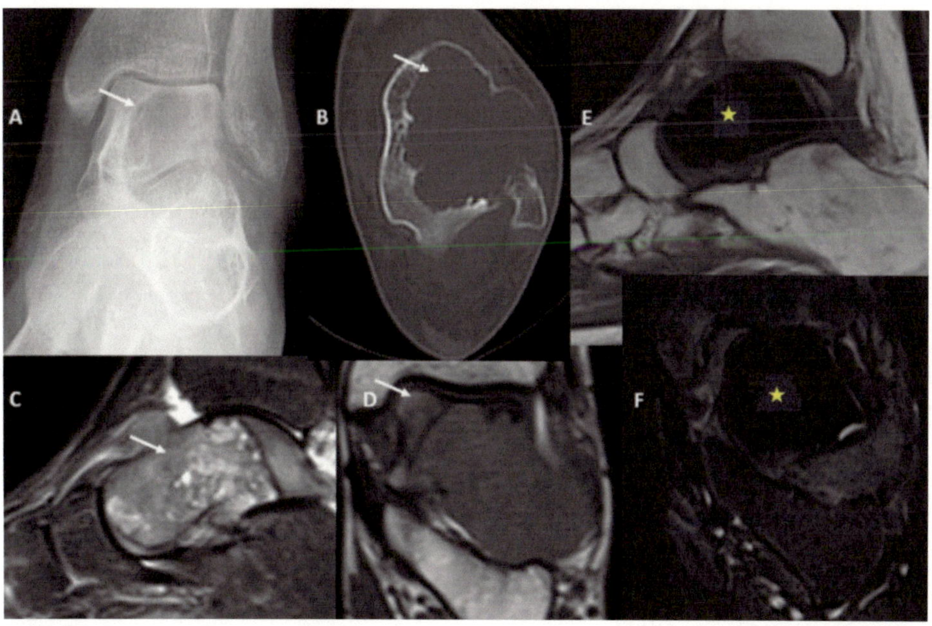

Figure 23.
Giant cell tumor: Frontal radiograph of the left ankle (A) demonstrates a circumscribed lytic lesion (white arrow) in the talus. Axial CT bone window image (B) better depicts the lobulated lytic lesion (white arrow) with scalloped margins. The lytic lesion (white arrow) demonstrates a heterogeneous hyperintense T2 signal (C). On the T1-weighted image (D), the lesion is isointense to muscle. Post-treatment MR images reveal dense hypointense signal on both T1-weighted (E) and T2-weighted (F).

3.3 Vascular lesions

3.3.1 Intraosseous hemangioma

Intraosseous hemangioma (IH) is a benign, slow-growing vascular neoplasm. Though it mainly involves the vertebrae and craniofacial bones, it can rarely involve long bones (mainly intramedullary in metadiaphyseal region; rarely cortical or subperiosteal) [79]. IH are usually identified in females between the age of 30–50 years. The most common pathologic type is cavernous hemangioma. On radiographs, intraosseous hemangiomas may show a "sunburst" or "honeycomb" appearance. On CT, IH may demonstrate the classic "polka dot" sign (due to associated coarse appearance of the trabecular bone), honeycomb appearance of the lytic lesion (because of internal linear trabeculations), or a spiculated "Irish lace" pattern. MRI helps in better delineation of location and extent of the hemangioma. On MRI, IH demonstrates intermediate to high T1 signal, high T2 signal, and diffuse or peripheral enhancement with signal intensity similar to the adjacent vessels [80] (**Figure 24A** and **B**). Most of the IH lesions are asymptomatic and need no treatment. Symptomatic vertebral hemangiomas without neurologic deficits can be managed by radiotherapy [81].

3.4 Tumor mimickers

1. **Brodie Abscess:** Brodie Abscess is an intraosseous abscess associated with subacute pyogenic osteomyelitis and can often be confused as a bone tumor. There is typically an insidious onset with systemic inflammatory signs, and symptoms are often absent [82]. *Staphylococcus aureus* is the most common organism involved. It typically occurs in the metaphysis of long bones, with proximal and distal tibial metaphyses are most commonly involved. On radiography/CT, Brodie abscess is typically a metaphyseal radiolucent lesion with a sclerotic rim along the long axis of the bone (**Figure 25A**). If a lucent

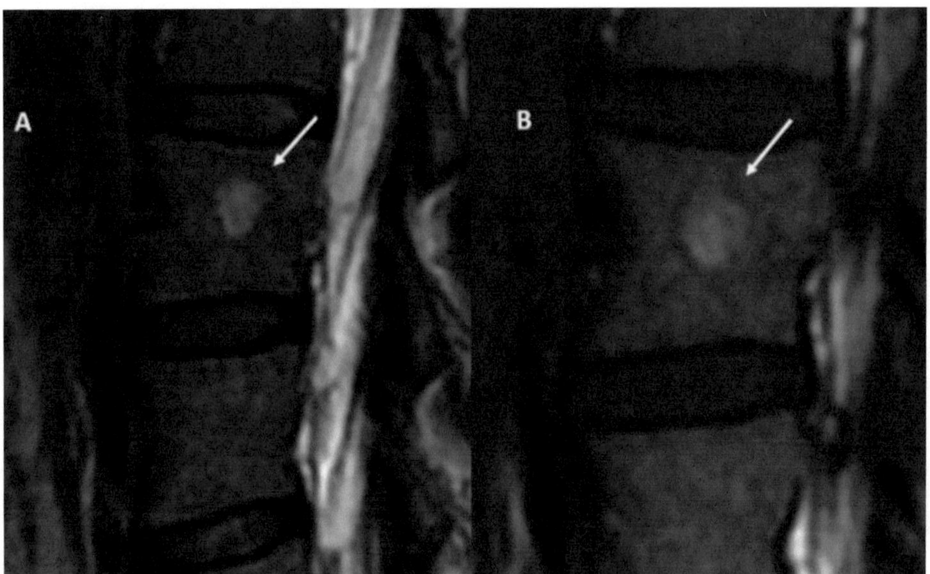

Figure 24.
Intraosseous hemangioma: Sagittal MR images of lumbar spine reveal a focal well-circumscribed signal abnormality in the vertebral body (white arrows) that is hyperintense on both T2-weighted (A) and T1-weighted (B) images represent a small vertebral hemangioma.

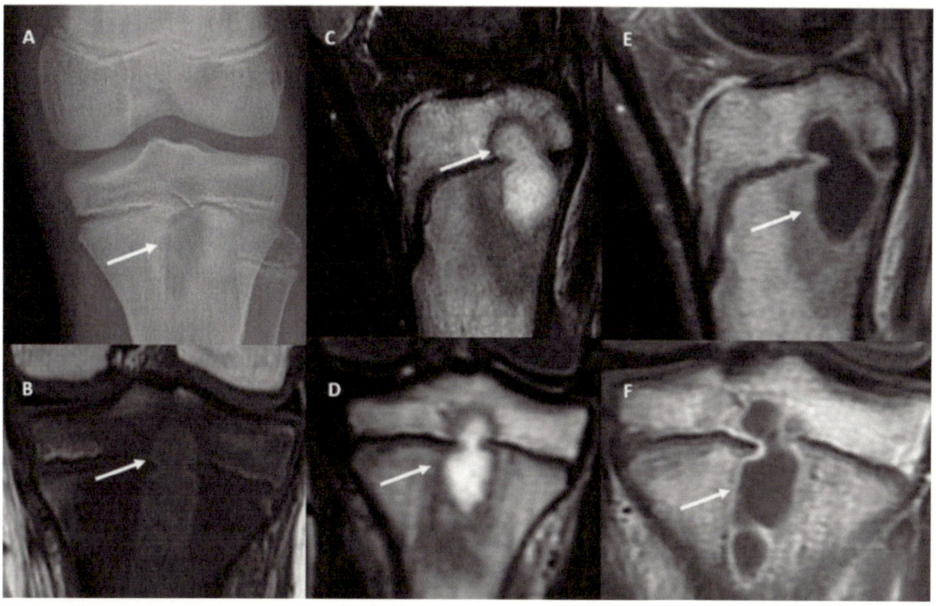

Figure 25.
Brodie Abscess: Frontal radiograph of the left knee (A) shows a lucent area (white arrow) with a faintly sclerotic peripheral rim in the proximal tibial epi-metaphyseal region. B demonstrates the "Penumbra sign" with rim lining of the abscess cavity (white arrow) with higher signal intensity than that of the remaining abscess on T1-weighted imaging. The abscess shows increased T2 signal (white arrows; C-D) and peripheral rim enhancement (white arrows) on the postcontrast images (E-F).

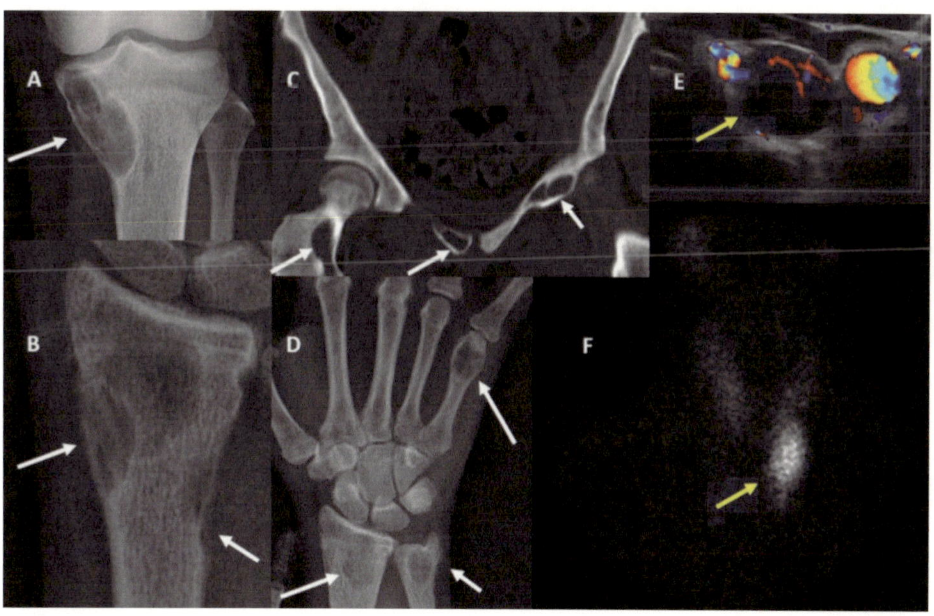

Figure 26.
Brown tumor: Frontal radiograph of the left knee (A) shows an eccentric, well-defined, lytic lesion (white arrow) in the proximal tibial epi-metaphyseal region with associated thinning and expansion of cortex. Similar appearing lytic areas (white arrows) are identified in the distal radius (B), pelvic bones and proximal right femur (C), and distal radius and ulna and proximal fifth metacarpal (D). Color flow ultrasound image of the neck (E) demonstrates a well-defined hypoechoic solid parathyroid mass (yellow arrow). The parathyroid mass appears as a hot spot (yellow arrow) on nuclear imaging scan (F).

tract extends to physis, diagnosis of Brodie abscess is strongly suggested. There may be associated periosteal reaction. On MRI, there is a T1 hypointense center with T1 hyperintense rim due to peripheral vascularized granulation tissue lining the abscess cavity, which is also termed as “MR penumbra sign” [83] (**Figure 25B–E**). There is typical rim enhancement following contrast administration (**Figure 25F**). Brodie abscess is usually treated with surgical curettage and antibiotic therapy [82].

2. **Brown Tumor/Osteitis Fibrosa Cystica:** Brown tumor, also known as osteitis fibrosa cystica is the skeletal manifestation of hyperparathyroidism, most commonly related to parathyroid adenoma. Parathormone induces osteoclastic activity, which results in multifocal bone cyst formation and osteopenia. The name brown tumor is derived from color resulting from hemosiderin deposition. Brown tumor is rare, seen in less than 3% of cases of hyperparathyroidism [84]. On radiography/CT, these lesions are typically multifocal well-defined radiolucent lesions with expansion and thinning of the overlying cortex (**Figure 26A–D**). SPECT or planar scintigraphy using Tc-99 m sestamibi shows high radiotracer uptake in parathyroid adenoma (**Figure 26F**). Fusion SPECT–CT can aid in further localization. Brown tumor usually resolves after treatment of hyperparathyroidism in the form of surgical resection of parathyroid adenoma or medical treatment depending on the cause.

Author details

Jignesh Shah* and Ankita Chauhan
Department of Pediatric Radiology, University of Tennessee Health Science Center, Memphis, Tennessee, United States

*Address all correspondence to: jshah3@uthsc.edu

References

[1] S. Noordin, S. Allana, M. Umer, M. Jamil, K. Hilal, and N. Uddin, "Unicameral bone cysts: Current concepts," Ann Med Surg (Lond), vol. 34, pp. 43-49, Oct 2018, doi: 10.1016/j.amsu.2018.06.005.

[2] E. Mascard, A. Gomez-Brouchet, and K. Lambot, "Bone cysts: Unicameral and aneurysmal bone cyst," Orthop Traumatol Surg Res, vol. 101, no. 1 Suppl, pp. S119-S127, Feb 2015, doi: 10.1016/j.otsr.2014.06.031.

[3] W. F. Jackson, T. N. Theologis, C. L. Gibbons, S. Mathews, and G. Kambouroglou, "Early management of pathological fractures in children," Injury, vol. 38, no. 2, pp. 194-200, Feb 2007, doi: 10.1016/j.injury.2006.07.040.

[4] M. S. Rosario *et al.*, "An unusual case of proximal humeral simple bone cyst in an adult from secondary cystic change," World J Surg Oncol, vol. 15, no. 1, p. 102, May 15 2017, doi: 10.1186/s12957-017-1166-8.

[5] J. N. Shah, H. L. Cohen, A. F. Choudhri, S. Gupta, and S. F. Miller, "Pediatric benign bone tumors: What does the radiologist need to know?: Pediatric imaging," Radiographics, vol. 37, no. 3, pp. 1001-1002, May-Jun 2017, doi: 10.1148/rg.2017160143.

[6] H. Aiba *et al.*, "Treatment of simple bone cysts using endoscopic curettage: A case series analysis," J Orthop Surg Res, vol. 13, no. 1, p. 168, Jul 5 2018, doi: 10.1186/s13018-018-0869-z.

[7] H. Y. Hou, K. Wu, C. T. Wang, S. M. Chang, W. H. Lin, and R. S. Yang, "Treatment of unicameral bone cyst: A comparative study of selected techniques," J Bone Joint Surg Am, vol. 92, no. 4, pp. 855-862, Apr 2010, doi: 10.2106/JBJS.I.00607.

[8] M. G. Weber, J. Fan, and R. Jenkins, "An Uncommon Presentation of an Uncommon Bone Tumor: A Case Study of a Pathologic Fracture of an Intertrochanteric Aneurysmal Bone Cyst," *Cureus*, vol. 11, no. 12, p. e6461, Dec 25 2019, doi: 10.7759/cureus.6461.

[9] F. Grahneis *et al.*, "Aneurysmal bone cyst: A review of 65 patients," J Bone Oncol, vol. 18, p. 100255, Oct 2019, doi: 10.1016/j.jbo.2019.100255.

[10] R. Capanna, D. A. Campanacci, and M. Manfrini, "Unicameral and aneurysmal bone cysts," *Orthop Clin North Am*, vol. 27, no. 3, pp. 605-14, Jul 1996. [Online]. Available: https://www.ncbi.nlm.nih.gov/pubmed/8649741.

[11] R. J. Sullivan, J. S. Meyer, J. P. Dormans, and R. S. Davidson, "Diagnosing aneurysmal and unicameral bone cysts with magnetic resonance imaging," *Clin Orthop Relat Res*, no. 366, pp. 186-90, Sep 1999, doi: 10.1097/00003086-199909000-00024.

[12] H. Y. Park *et al.*, "Current management of aneurysmal bone cysts," Curr Rev Musculoskelet Med, vol. 9, no. 4, pp. 435-444, Dec 2016, doi: 10.1007/s12178-016-9371-6.

[13] L. B. Gutierrez, T. M. Link, A. E. Horvai, G. B. Joseph, R. J. O'Donnell, and D. Motamedi, "Secondary aneurysmal bone cysts and associated primary lesions: Imaging features of 49 cases," Clin Imaging, vol. 62, pp. 23-32, Jun 2020, doi: 10.1016/j.clinimag.2020.01.022.

[14] P. P. Lin, C. Brown, A. K. Raymond, M. T. Deavers, and A. W. Yasko, "Aneurysmal bone cysts recur at juxtaphyseal locations in skeletally immature patients," Clin Orthop Relat Res, vol. 466, no. 3, pp. 722-728,

Mar 2008, doi: 10.1007/s11999-007-0080-8.

[15] P. Tsagozis and O. Brosjo, "Current Strategies for the Treatment of Aneurysmal Bone Cysts," *Orthop Rev (Pavia),* vol. 7, no. 4, p. 6182, Dec 28 2015, doi: 10.4081/or.2015.6182.

[16] T. T. Nguyen, J. C. Thelen, and A. A. Bhatt, "Bone up on spinal osseous lesions: A case review series," Insights Imaging, vol. 11, no. 1, p. 80, Jun 29 2020, doi: 10.1186/s13244-020-00883-6.

[17] N. A. Avila, A. J. Dwyer, A. Rabel, T. Darling, C. H. Hong, and J. Moss, "CT of sclerotic bone lesions: Imaging features differentiating tuberous sclerosis complex with lymphangioleiomyomatosis from sporadic lymphangioleiomymatosis," Radiology, vol. 254, no. 3, pp. 851-857, Mar 2010, doi: 10.1148/radiol.09090227.

[18] A. Ulano *et al.*, "Distinguishing untreated osteoblastic metastases from Enostoses using CT attenuation measurements," AJR Am J Roentgenol, vol. 207, no. 2, pp. 362-368, Aug 2016, doi: 10.2214/AJR.15.15559.

[19] S. Bernard, E. Walker, and M. Raghavan, "An approach to the evaluation of incidentally identified bone lesions encountered on imaging studies," AJR Am J Roentgenol, vol. 208, no. 5, pp. 960-970, May 2017, doi: 10.2214/AJR.16.17434.

[20] G. P. Nielsen and A. E. Rosenberg, "Update on bone forming tumors of the head and neck," Head Neck Pathol, vol. 1, no. 1, pp. 87-93, Sep 2007, doi: 10.1007/s12105-007-0023-4.

[21] L. M. Lehmer, P. Kissel, and B. D. Ragsdale, "Frontal sinus osteoma with osteoblastoma-like histology and associated intracranial pneumatocele," Head Neck Pathol, vol. 6, no. 3, pp. 384-388, Sep 2012, doi: 10.1007/s12105-012-0332-0.

[22] A. G. Chiu, I. Schipor, N. A. Cohen, D. W. Kennedy, and J. N. Palmer, "Surgical decisions in the management of frontal sinus osteomas," *Am J Rhinol,* vol. 19, no. 2, pp. 191-7, Mar-Apr 2005. [Online]. Available: https://www.ncbi.nlm.nih.gov/pubmed/15921220.

[23] A. Rokade and A. Sama, "Update on management of frontal sinus osteomas," Curr Opin Otolaryngol Head Neck Surg, vol. 20, no. 1, pp. 40-44, Feb 2012, doi: 10.1097/MOO.0b013e32834e9037.

[24] M. R. Baruffi, J. B. Volpon, J. B. Neto, and C. Casartelli, "Osteoid osteomas with chromosome alterations involving 22q," *Cancer Genet Cytogenet,* vol. 124, no. 2, pp. 127-31, Jan 15 2001, doi: 10.1016/s0165-4608(00)00327-7.

[25] S. Noordin *et al.*, "Osteoid osteoma: Contemporary management," *Orthop Rev (Pavia),* vol. 10, no. 3, p. 7496, Sep 5 2018, doi: 10.4081/or.2018.7496.

[26] K. Motamedi and L. L. Seeger, "Benign bone tumors," *Radiol Clin North Am,* vol. 49, no. 6, pp. 1115-34, v, Nov 2011, doi: 10.1016/j.rcl.2011.07.002.

[27] A. Saifuddin, J. White, Z. Sherazi, M. I. Shaikh, C. Natali, and A. O. Ransford, "Osteoid osteoma and osteoblastoma of the spine. Factors associated with the presence of scoliosis," *Spine (Phila Pa 1976),* vol. 23, no. 1, pp. 47-53, Jan 1 1998, doi: 10.1097/00007632-199801010-00010.

[28] B. C. Carneiro *et al.*, "Osteoid osteoma: the great mimicker," *Insights Imaging,* vol. 12, no. 1, p. 32, Mar 8 2021, doi: 10.1186/s13244-021-00978-8.

[29] J. W. Chai *et al.*, "Radiologic diagnosis of osteoid osteoma: From simple to challenging findings," Radiographics, vol. 30, no. 3, pp. 737-749, May 2010, doi: 10.1148/rg.303095120.

[30] A. Chahal, P. Rajalakshmi, S. A. Khan, S. Rastogi, D. N. Srivastava, and S. Gamanagatti, "CT-guided percutaneous radiofrequency ablation of osteoid osteoma: Our experience in 87 patients," Indian J Radiol Imaging, vol. 27, no. 2, pp. 207-215, Apr-Jun 2017, doi: 10.4103/ijri.IJRI_260_16.

[31] M. A. Galgano, C. R. Goulart, H. Iwenofu, L. S. Chin, W. Lavelle, and E. Mendel, "Osteoblastomas of the spine: A comprehensive review," Neurosurg Focus, vol. 41, no. 2, p. E4, Aug 2016, doi: 10.3171/2016.5.FOCUS16122.

[32] P. K. Avadhanam, S. Vuyyur, and M. K. Panigrahi, "A rare occurrence of osteoblastoma in a child," J Pediatr Neurosci, vol. 5, no. 2, pp. 153-156, Jul 2010, doi: 10.4103/1817-1745.76118.

[33] M. Wu *et al.*, "Diagnostic and management options of Osteoblastoma in the spine," Med Sci Monit, vol. 25, pp. 1362-1372, Feb 20 2019, doi: 10.12659/MSM.913666.

[34] A. Honda *et al.*, "Recurrent lumbar-origin osteoblastoma treated with multiple surgery and carbon ion radiotherapy: A case report," BMC Musculoskelet Disord, vol. 21, no. 1, p. 321, May 22 2020, doi: 10.1186/s12891-020-03349-4.

[35] Z. Huang *et al.*, "Imaging algorithm and multimodality evaluation of spinal osteoblastoma," *BMC Musculoskelet Disord,* vol. 21, no. 1, p. 240, Apr 14 2020, doi: 10.1186/s12891-020-03252-y.

[36] A. L. Versteeg *et al.*, "Surgical management of spinal osteoblastomas," J Neurosurg Spine, vol. 27, no. 3, pp. 321-327, Sep 2017, doi: 10.3171/2017.1.SPINE16788.

[37] B. D. Elder *et al.*, "Surgical Management of Osteoblastoma of the spine: Case series and review of the literature," Turk Neurosurg, vol. 26, no. 4, pp. 601-607, 2016, doi: 10.5137/1019-5149.JTN.14348-15.1.

[38] C. T. Kraft, R. J. Morrison, and H. A. Arts, "Malignant transformation of a high-grade osteoblastoma of the petrous apex with subcutaneous metastasis," *Ear Nose Throat J,* vol. 95, no. 6, pp. 230-3, Jun 2016. [Online]. Available: https://www.ncbi.nlm.nih.gov/pubmed/27304442.

[39] M. J. Walden, M. D. Murphey, and J. A. Vidal, "Incidental enchondromas of the knee," AJR Am J Roentgenol, vol. 190, no. 6, pp. 1611-1615, Jun 2008, doi: 10.2214/AJR.07.2796.

[40] T. Reisler, S. L. Viviano, and M. Granick, "Osseous tumor of the hand: finger enchondroma," *Eplasty,* vol. 15, p. ic4, 2015. [Online]. Available: https://www.ncbi.nlm.nih.gov/pubmed/25671055.

[41] S. Capkin, A. Cavit, K. Yilmaz, and T. Kaleli, "Surgical Treatment of Solitary Enchondromas of the Hand," *Cureus,* vol. 12, no. 4, p. e7497, Apr 1 2020, doi: 10.7759/cureus.7497.

[42] T. De Coninck *et al.*, "Dynamic contrast-enhanced MR imaging for differentiation between enchondroma and chondrosarcoma," Eur Radiol, vol. 23, no. 11, pp. 3140-3152, Nov 2013, doi: 10.1007/s00330-013-2913-z.

[43] C. Silve and H. Juppner, "Ollier disease," Orphanet J Rare Dis, vol. 1, p. 37, Sep 22 2006, doi: 10.1186/1750-1172-1-37.

[44] T. C. Pansuriya, H. M. Kroon, and J. V. Bovee, "Enchondromatosis: insights on the different subtypes," *Int J Clin Exp Pathol,* vol. 3, no. 6, pp. 557-69, Jun 26 2010. [Online]. Available: https://www.ncbi.nlm.nih.gov/pubmed/20661403.

[45] J. Yang, W. Tian, X. Zhu, and J. Wang, "Chondroblastoma in the long

bone diaphysis: A report of two cases with literature review," Chin J Cancer, vol. 31, no. 5, pp. 257-264, May 2012, doi: 10.5732/cjc.011.10402.

[46] S. J. Swarts, J. R. Neff, S. L. Johansson, M. Nelson, and J. A. Bridge, "Significance of abnormalities of chromosomes 5 and 8 in chondroblastoma," *Clin Orthop Relat Res,* no. 349, pp. 189-93, Apr 1998, doi: 10.1097/00003086-199804000-00023.

[47] W. Chen and L. M. DiFrancesco, "Chondroblastoma: An Update," Arch Pathol Lab Med, vol. 141, no. 6, pp. 867-871, Jun 2017, doi: 10.5858/arpa.2016-0281-RS.

[48] P. T. Weatherall, G. E. Maale, D. B. Mendelsohn, C. S. Sherry, W. E. Erdman, and H. R. Pascoe, "Chondroblastoma: Classic and confusing appearance at MR imaging," Radiology, vol. 190, no. 2, pp. 467-474, Feb 1994, doi: 10.1148/radiology.190.2.8284401.

[49] S. Cappelle, S. Pans, and R. Sciot, "Imaging features of chondromyxoid fibroma: Report of 15 cases and literature review," Br J Radiol, vol. 89, no. 1064, p. 20160088, Aug 2016, doi: 10.1259/bjr.20160088.

[50] H. S. Kim *et al.*, "MRI of chondromyxoid fibroma," *Acta Radiol,* vol. 52, no. 8, pp. 875-80, Oct 1 2011, doi: 10.1258/ar.2011.110180.

[51] J. S. Bhamra *et al.*, "Chondromyxoid fibroma management: A single institution experience of 22 cases," World J Surg Oncol, vol. 12, p. 283, Sep 12 2014, doi: 10.1186/1477-7819-12-283.

[52] K. Tepelenis *et al.*, "Osteochondromas: An updated review of epidemiology, pathogenesis, clinical presentation, radiological features and treatment options," In Vivo, vol. 35, no. 2, pp. 681-691, Mar-Apr 2021, doi: 10.21873/invivo.12308.

[53] A. M. de Souza and R. Z. Bispo Junior, "Osteochondroma: ignore or investigate?," *Rev Bras Ortop,* vol. 49, no. 6, pp. 555-64, Nov-Dec 2014, doi: 10.1016/j.rboe.2013.10.002.

[54] M. D. Murphey, J. J. Choi, M. J. Kransdorf, D. J. Flemming, and F. H. Gannon, "Imaging of osteochondroma: Variants and complications with radiologic-pathologic correlation," Radiographics, vol. 20, no. 5, pp. 1407-1434, Sep-Oct 2000, doi: 10.1148/radiographics.20.5.g00se171407.

[55] J. V. Bovee, "Multiple osteochondromas," Orphanet J Rare Dis, vol. 3, p. 3, Feb 13 2008, doi: 10.1186/1750-1172-3-3.

[56] C. M. Czajka and M. R. DiCaprio, "What is the proportion of patients with multiple hereditary exostoses who undergo malignant degeneration?," Clin Orthop Relat Res, vol. 473, no. 7, pp. 2355-2361, Jul 2015, doi: 10.1007/s11999-015-4134-z.

[57] A. J. Degnan and V. M. Ho-Fung, "More than epiphyseal Osteochondromas: Updated understanding of imaging findings in dysplasia Epiphysealis Hemimelica (Trevor disease)," AJR Am J Roentgenol, vol. 211, no. 4, pp. 910-919, Oct 2018, doi: 10.2214/AJR.18.19712.

[58] L. A. Semenova and I. V. Bulycheva, "[Chondromas (enchondroma, periosteal chondroma, enchondromatosis)]," *Arkh Patol,* vol. 69, no. 5, pp. 45-8, Sep-Oct 2007. [Online]. Available: https://www.ncbi.nlm.nih.gov/pubmed/18074822.

[59] P. Robinson *et al.*, "Periosteal chondroid tumors: Radiologic evaluation with pathologic correlation," AJR Am J Roentgenol, vol. 177, no. 5, pp. 1183-1188, Nov 2001, doi: 10.2214/ajr.177.5.1771183.

[60] M. Blaz, P. Palczewski, J. Swiatkowski, and M. Golebiowski, "Cortical fibrous defects and non-ossifying fibromas in children and young adults: The analysis of radiological features in 28 cases and a review of literature," *Pol J Radiol,* vol. 76, no. 4, pp. 32-9, Oct 2011. [Online]. Available: https://www.ncbi.nlm.nih.gov/pubmed/22802852.

[61] G. S. Goodin, B. L. Shulkin, R. A. Kaufman, and M. B. McCarville, "PET/CT characterization of fibroosseous defects in children: 18F-FDG uptake can mimic metastatic disease," AJR Am J Roentgenol, vol. 187, no. 4, pp. 1124-1128, Oct 2006, doi: 10.2214/AJR.06.0171.

[62] L. M. Bowers, D. M. Cohen, I. Bhattacharyya, J. C. Pettigrew, Jr., and M. F. Stavropoulos, "The non-ossifying fibroma: A case report and review of the literature," Head Neck Pathol, vol. 7, no. 2, pp. 203-210, Jun 2013, doi: 10.1007/s12105-012-0399-7.

[63] K. Jamshidi, P. Motaghi, A. Bagherifard, M. Eigi, H. H. Al-Bascesee, and A. Mirzaei, "Comparison of Characteristic Features and Local Recurrence in Syndromic Versus Non-syndromic Multifocal Non-ossifying Fibroma," *J Orthop Sci,* Aug 17 2020, doi: 10.1016/j.jos.2020.06.010.

[64] A. R. Kinnunen, R. Sironen, and P. Sipola, "Magnetic resonance imaging characteristics in patients with histopathologically proven fibrous dysplasia-a systematic review," Skeletal Radiol, vol. 49, no. 6, pp. 837-845, Jun 2020, doi: 10.1007/s00256-020-03388-x.

[65] E. Gokce and M. Beyhan, "Radiological imaging findings of craniofacial fibrous dysplasia," Turk Neurosurg, vol. 30, no. 6, pp. 799-807, 2020, doi: 10.5137/1019-5149.JTN.24627-18.2.

[66] M. Wilson and C. Snyderman, "Fibro-osseous lesions of the Skull Base in the pediatric population," J Neurol Surg B Skull Base, vol. 79, no. 1, pp. 31-36, Feb 2018, doi: 10.1055/s-0037-1617440.

[67] M. K. Javaid *et al.*, "Best practice management guidelines for fibrous dysplasia/McCune-Albright syndrome: A consensus statement from the FD/MAS international consortium," Orphanet J Rare Dis, vol. 14, no. 1, p. 139, Jun 13 2019, doi: 10.1186/s13023-019-1102-9.

[68] A. Butt, K. Patel, K. Agrawal, A. Arya, and J. Singh, "Fibrous dysplasia of the clivus - a case study and literature review," Radiol Case Rep, vol. 16, no. 2, pp. 230-236, Feb 2021, doi: 10.1016/j.radcr.2020.11.019.

[69] D. Franz *et al.*, "Milk cloud appearance-a characteristic sign of fibrous dysplasia on contrast-enhanced MR imaging," Eur Radiol, vol. 29, no. 7, pp. 3424-3430, Jul 2019, doi: 10.1007/s00330-019-06245-1.

[70] G. Z. Papadakis *et al.*, "(18) F-NaF PET/CT IMAGING IN FIBROUS DYSPLASIA OF BONE," J Bone Miner Res, vol. 34, no. 9, pp. 1619-1631, Sep 2019, doi: 10.1002/jbmr.3738.

[71] R. Chapurlat and M. A. Legrand, "Bisphosphonates for the treatment of fibrous dysplasia of bone," Bone, vol. 143, p. 115784, Feb 2021, doi: 10.1016/j.bone.2020.115784.

[72] H. Park, M. Nishino, J. L. Hornick, and E. D. Jacobsen, "Imaging of Histiocytosis in the era of genomic medicine," Radiographics, vol. 39, no. 1, pp. 95-114, Jan-Feb 2019, doi: 10.1148/rg.2019180054.

[73] J. Zaveri, Q. La, G. Yarmish, and J. Neuman, "More than just Langerhans cell histiocytosis: A radiologic review of histiocytic disorders," Radiographics,

vol. 34, no. 7, pp. 2008-2024, Nov-Dec 2014, doi: 10.1148/rg.347130132.

[74] C. J. Chakarun, D. M. Forrester, C. J. Gottsegen, D. B. Patel, E. A. White, and G. R. Matcuk, Jr., "Giant cell tumor of bone: Review, mimics, and new developments in treatment," Radiographics, vol. 33, no. 1, pp. 197-211, Jan-Feb 2013, doi: 10.1148/rg.331125089.

[75] H. M. Pereira, E. Marchiori, and A. Severo, "Magnetic resonance imaging aspects of giant-cell tumours of bone," J Med Imaging Radiat Oncol, vol. 58, no. 6, pp. 674-678, Dec 2014, doi: 10.1111/1754-9485.12249.

[76] L. S. Shi, Y. Q. Li, W. J. Wu, Z. K. Zhang, F. Gao, and M. Latif, "Imaging appearance of giant cell tumour of the spine above the sacrum," Br J Radiol, vol. 88, no. 1051, p. 20140566, Jul 2015, doi: 10.1259/bjr.20140566.

[77] Y. He *et al.*, "Magnetic resonance feature of "paintbrush borders" sign as a novel way to predict recurrence of giant cell tumor of bone after curettage: A pilot study," J Int Med Res, vol. 46, no. 2, pp. 710-722, Feb 2018, doi: 10.1177/0300060517720345.

[78] L. van der Heijden *et al.*, "The clinical approach toward giant cell tumor of bone," *Oncologist,* vol. 19, no. 5, pp. 550-61, May 2014, doi: 10.1634/theoncologist.2013-0432.

[79] A. Rigopoulou and A. Saifuddin, "Intraosseous hemangioma of the appendicular skeleton: Imaging features of 15 cases, and a review of the literature," Skeletal Radiol, vol. 41, no. 12, pp. 1525-1536, Dec 2012, doi: 10.1007/s00256-012-1444-z.

[80] Q. Zhou, L. Lu, Z. Yang, S. Su, and G. Hong, "Hemangioma of long tubular bone: Imaging characteristics with emphasis on magnetic resonance imaging," Skeletal Radiol, vol. 49, no. 12, pp. 2029-2038, Dec 2020, doi: 10.1007/s00256-020-03527-4.

[81] K. Yao, F. Tang, L. Min, Y. Zhou, and C. Tu, "Multifocal intraosseous hemangioma: A case report," *Medicine (Baltimore),* vol. 98, no. 2, p. e14001, Jan 2019, doi: 10.1097/MD.0000000000014001.

[82] N. van der Naald, D. P. J. Smeeing, R. M. Houwert, F. Hietbrink, G. A. M. Govaert, and D. van der Velde, "Brodie's abscess: A systematic review of reported cases," J Bone Jt Infect, vol. 4, no. 1, pp. 33-39, 2019, doi: 10.7150/jbji.31843.

[83] A. Afshar and A. Mohammadi, "The "penumbra sign" on magnetic resonance images of Brodie's abscess: A case report," Iran J Radiol, vol. 8, no. 4, pp. 245-248, Dec 2011, doi: 10.5812/iranjradiol.4493.

[84] C. Xie, M. Tsakok, N. Taylor, and K. Partington, "Imaging of brown tumours: A pictorial review," Insights Imaging, vol. 10, no. 1, p. 75, Jul 29 2019, doi: 10.1186/s13244-019-0757-z.

Chapter 3

Medical Therapy of Giant Cell Tumor of Bone

Raquel Lopes-Brás, Isabel Fernandes, Sandra Casimiro and Luís Costa

Abstract

Giant cell tumor of bone (GCTB) is mostly a benign disease of the bone, although with high local recurrence rate and potential for metastatic spread, namely to the lungs. It is also a locally aggressive tumor, associated with severe morbidity and functional impairment due to bone destruction. Treatment is therefore required and should be offered at an early stage to allow complete resection, minimizing functional sequelae and local recurrence. Surgical resection is the mainstay of treatment, often followed by intralesional adjuvant therapy. GCTB has a particular biology, in which RANKL represents a key factor in tumor pathogenesis, thus making this molecule a valuable therapeutic target. Monthly administration of denosumab, a fully human monoclonal antibody directed against RANKL, has been studied in several clinical trials and shown a high rate of local control with favorable safety profile. In this chapter, current medical management, ongoing studies, and future directions in GCTB will be discussed.

Keywords: denosumab, giant cell tumor of bone, RANKL, sarcoma, sarcomatoid transformation

1. Introduction

Giant cell tumor of bone (GCTB) is a primary tumor of bone usually arising in the meta-epiphysis of long bones, although potentially also occur in other parts of the skeleton, such as the spine or pelvis [1]. GCTB more often affects young patients in the second to forth decades of life [1, 2] and those living in urban (rather than rural) areas [3]. It is also associated with Paget's disease [4]. The condition presents with localized pain, tenderness to touch, palpable mass, and decreased range of motion, as well as mechanical pain and joint swelling in patients with presentation near joints [5]. Rarely, it may present with pathological fracture [4].

GCTB is mostly a benign disease, but local recurrence rates are high and there is a small risk of metastatic spread, namely to the lungs [1, 6]. Risk factors for pulmonary metastases include young age, Enneking stage 3, local recurrence, and axial disease, but not treatment modality [6, 7]. Pulmonary metastases most often appear three to four years after initial diagnosis and rarely are the cause of death [8]. However, when GCTB metastasizes, mortality rate rises to 14–25% [8, 9].

Despite being a rare event, GCTB can also undergo malignant sarcomatoid transformation [10]. In these cases, malignant GCTB can present with three histologic subtypes: osteosarcoma, fibrosarcoma, or undifferentiated pleomorphic sarcoma. This usually occurs following multiple recurrent lesions (e.g. Paget's disease) and/or radiation therapy [5].

Multicentric GCTB in another rare form of tumor presentation, characterized by two or more distant lesions of histologically confirmed disease [11]. These lesions can present as synchronous (more common) or metachronous. Although multicentric GCTB appears to have demographic differences (patients are young and more commonly female), disease behavior – including local recurrence rates, pulmonary metastases pattern, and malignant transformation – seems to be similar to solitary GCTB [11].

Radiologically, GCTB presents as an osteolytic lesion with characteristic radiolucent and geographic (well-circumscribed) appearance and fading cortical bone, rarely showing periosteal reaction. GCTBs are usually eccentric masses in the epiphyseal region extending to subchondral bone (sclerotic metaphyseal margin) [5, 12].

Besides a high degree of suspicion in radiological exams (plain films, computed tomography [CT], and magnetic resonance imaging [MRI]), GCTB diagnosis must be histologically confirmed by core-needle or open biopsy [5]. Still, plain radiographs, CT scan, and MRI are useful for diagnosis and local staging. MRI is often performed to delineate neoplasm extent, namely soft tissue extension. Additionally, bone scintigraphy helps ruling out other asymptomatic bone lesions and chest CT scan should be performed to exclude lung involvement and guide treatment.

Based on radiological findings and according to Enneking and later Campanacci grading systems, GCTB can be classified in three grades [7, 13]:

- Grade I (latent): well-defined margin (thin rim of mature bone) and intact cortex (not deformed).

- Grade II (active): relatively well-defined margins but no radiopaque rim; cortex is thinned and moderately expanded. Grade II lesions with fracture are graded separately.

- Grade II (aggressive): indistinct borders and cortex destruction, suggesting rapid and permeated growth.

This surgical staging system allows preoperative planning. Post-operatively, GCTB can also be graded based on histological features in grade 1 (typical), grade 2 (aggressive), or grade 3 (malignant) [14].

Due to lack of long-term follow-up data, GCTB prognosis is not well established to date [15]. However, the overall prognosis of benign GCTB is generally favorable. Recurrence rates are estimated at 25% [15] and can be as high as 50% after curettage alone [16]. Systemic treatment with bisphosphonates or denosumab seems to lower these figures [17]. Although secondary lung involvement is rare in benign GCTB and very uncommonly the cause of death, mortality rate is higher in these patients (14–25%) [8, 9, 18]. Regarding malignant GCTB (either primary or secondary), overall survival at 5 years is about 85% and poorest in older patients and those with distant disease at diagnosis, according to a Surveillance, Epidemiology and End Results (SEER) study involving 117 cases of malignant GCTB [19]. Smaller studies may indicate worse survival rates [20].

2. GCTB biology and pathogenesis

2.1 Histopathology

GCTB is histologically characterized by diffuse growth of receptor activator of nuclear factor kappa-B ligand (RANKL)-positive, round-to-oval polygonal or elongated mononuclear stromal cells, RANK-positive mononuclear cells of myeloid linage, and RANK-positive osteoclast-like giant cells, reflecting a physiopathology intimately linked to the RANKL/RANK pathway [17, 21, 22] (**Figure 1**). Small areas of osteoid matrix deposition, woven bone, and occasionally new bone are also observed in about 50% of GCTB samples, with different studies reporting an incidence between 22 and 52% [23].

The characteristic giant cells in GCTB are osteoclastic in nature [24–28] and represent the reactive component responsible for GCTB aggressive lytic behavior, leading to GCTB designation as osteoclastoma. These cells express RANK but not RANKL [26]. Profiling studies have shown that giant cells in GCTB are the result of CD33+ pre-osteoclast fusion that further fuse with CD14+ mononuclear cells [27] and express tartrate-resistant acid phosphatase (TRAP) and vitronectin receptor, osteoclast markers, being capable of lacunar resorption [29].

However, in GCTB neoplastic cells are ovoid stromal cells, displaying markers of mesenchymal stem cells derived from the osteoblast lineage, but minimal expression of fully differentiated osteoblasts, like osteocalcin, alkaline phosphatase, osteoprotegerin (OPG), and TRAIL [29–33]. Twist-mediated downregulation of RUNX2, a major osteogenic regulator, has been shown to interrupt osteoblastic differentiation and depress osteoblast lineage markers in GCTB [34].

GCTB stromal cells express high levels of RANKL [27] and also produce other osteoclastogenic cytokines, like interleukin (IL)-1, −6, −11, and − 17, tumor necrosis factor-alpha (TNF-α), and macrophage colony-stimulating factor (M-CSF), through which osteoclast differentiation is stimulated from precursor cells [26]. Other characteristics supporting their neoplastic nature include dominance, increased proliferative potential, abundance of genetic alterations, and expression of more differentiation markers than multinucleated giant cells [22]. GCTBs are polyclonal in nature, with inconsistent chromosomal changes and telomere associations occurring in up to 72% of cases, although lacking prognostic value [35–38]. Mononuclear stromal cell-exclusive mutation p.G34W (or p.G34L, p.G34M, p. G34R, or p.G34V in a small sub-set of cases) in the *H3F3A* gene, encoding histone 3.3 (H3.3) variant implicated in epigenetic reprogramming and memory, has been identified as GCTB-specific driver mutation [30].

Because G34W mutations occur more frequently than chromosomal abnormalities and can be causative risk factors for chromosomal structural remodeling in DNA synthesis, it has been hypothesized that this driver mutation causes chromosomal instability and defects, contributing to pleiotropic effects on cell cycle-related expression, immature osteoblastic differentiation, and chemokines, cytokines, and

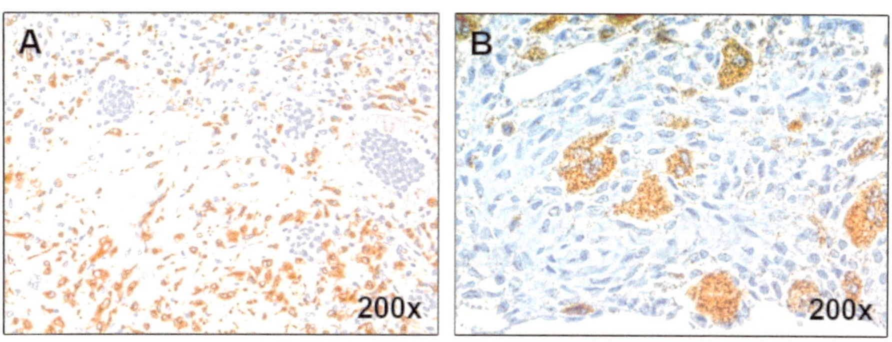

Figure 1.
Representative images of RANKL (A) and RANK (B) immunohistochemistry in formalin-fixed and paraffin-embedded GCTB samples. (unpublished data).

surface markers expression [22, 37]. Additionally, mutations in cyclin D1, p53, and MET have been linked to malignant transformation and GCTB recurrence [22].

Biologically, Wnt/β-catenin and transforming growth factor beta (TGF-β) signaling pathways mediate the exacerbated proliferation of stromal cells in GCTB. β-catenin, cyclin D1, and p21 have been shown to be overexpressed in the nuclei of GCTB stromal cells [39]. Additionally, one study showed that protease activated receptor-1 (PAR-1) is also upregulated in GCTB downstream of TGF-β, via Smad3 and Smad4 [40]. In the study, PAR-1 knockout in GCTB stromal cells inhibited tumor growth, angiogenesis, and osteoclastogenesis in vitro and PAR-1 inhibition suppressed tumor growth and giant cell formation *in vivo*.

2.2 Physiopathology

GCTB physiopathology is not entirely understood, but there is compelling evidence that RANKL overexpression by mononuclear stromal cells plays a key role and elicits transformation of monocytic pre-osteoclast to osteoclast cells, ultimately resulting in osteolysis observed in these tumors [22, 41–43] (**Figure 2**). Accordingly, preclinical models have shown that OPG, a soluble decoy receptor for RANKL, inhibits monocyte activation and osteoclast differentiation [44].

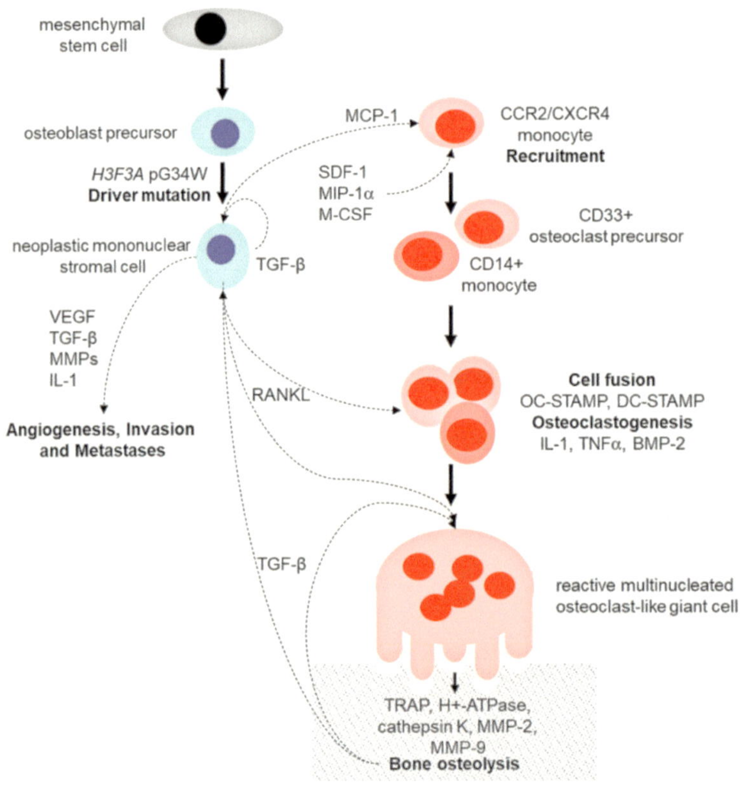

Figure 2.
Simplified scheme of GCTB physiopathology. BMP-2, bone morphogenetic protein 2; CCR2, C-C chemokine receptor type 2; CXCR4, C-X-C chemokine receptor type 4; DC-STAMP, dendritic cell-specific transmembrane protein; IL-1, interleukin 1; MCP-1, monocyte chemoattractant protein-1; M-CSF, macrophage colony-stimulating factor; MIP-1α, macrophage inflammatory protein 1-alpha; MMPs, matrix metalloproteases; OC-STAMP, osteoclast stimulatory transmembrane protein; RANKL, receptor activator of nuclear factor kappa-B ligand; SDF-1, stromal cell-derived factor 1; TGF-β, transforming growth factor beta; TNFα, tumor necrosis factor alpha; TRAP, tartrate-resistant acid phosphatase; VEGF, vascular endothelial growth factor.

In GCTB, stromal cell-derived monocyte chemoattractant protein-1 (MCP-1/CCL2) recruits bone marrow-derived CCR2/CXCR4-expressing monocytic osteoclast precursors from peripheral blood [45, 46]. Other soluble factors within GCTB microenvironment are chemotactic for myelomonocytic cells, including stromal cell-derived factor 1 (SDF-1/CXCL12), macrophage inflammatory protein 1-alpha (MIP-1α/CCL3), and M-CSF1 [26, 47]. Osteoclast precursors localized at GCTB microenvironment differentiate into active, bone resorbing, osteoclasts.

Different pre-clinical studies have shown that GCTB stromal cells with circulating mononuclear cells co-culture induces differentiation of osteolytic giant cells [41–43]. For differentiation to occur, RANKL expression in stromal cells is regulated by CCAAT/enhancer-binding protein beta (C/EBPβ), found to be overexpressed in GCTB [48], and also by parathyroid hormone-related peptide (PTHrP) in an autocrine manner [49]. Next, RANKL-induced cell fusion is co-stimulated by M-CSF and IL-34 [26] and enhanced by specific transmembrane proteins overexpressed in GCTB [50] and coupling components, like insulin-like growth factors (IGF) I and II [51].

RANK pathway activation in giant cells leads to up-regulation of nuclear factor of activated T cells c1 (NFATc1), an auto-regulated key transcription factor responsible for regulating expression of important genes involved in bone resorption, like cathepsin K or β3-integrin [52]. Cathepsin K is involved in initial steps of bone resorption, degrading collagen type I and remodeling the bone matrix, allowing migration. As bone resorption starts, TGF-β entrapped in bone matrix is activated by matrix metalloproteases (MMPs), stimulating giant cell migration [46], which is mediated by αvβ3 integrin attachment to the bone matrix [53].

MMPs have an important role in GCTB physiopathology. Apart from the above-mentioned role in giant cell migration via TGF-β activation, MMPs influence other major aspects within the tumor microenvironment, like angiogenesis, invasion, and metastatic development. MMP-2 and MMP-9 are key in all these processes [22]. In GCTB, the extracellular matrix metalloproteinase inducer (EMMPRIN) is responsible for inducing MMP expression. Higher EMMPRIN expression at multinuclear osteoclast-like giant cells has been observed in stage III GCTB, probably regulated by RANKL from stromal-like tumor cells [54].

As previously mentioned, metastases are extremely rare in GCTB and there are no clues on molecular or physiopathological events related with GCTB metastization to date.

2.3 Tumor markers

Pathophysiology of GCTB progression remains unclear and prognostic factors, treatment targets, and predictive biomarkers represent unmet needs.

Histologically, ambiguous giant cell-rich lesions – including benign GCTB, chondroblastoma, aneurysmal bone cyst, central giant cell granuloma of the jaw, and malignant giant cell–rich osteosarcoma – are often found, especially as small biopsy or curettage specimens [22]. In these cases, *H3F3A* gene p.G34W mutation can be used in the differential diagnosis, as it is almost GCTB-exclusive [30, 55]. Approximately 90% of GCTBs display the p.G34W mutation, with minor subsets (<2%) displaying p.G34L, p.G34M, p.G34R, or p.G34V variants. H3F3B p.K36M is the H3.3 mutation found in the vast majority (90–95%) of chondroblastomas [30].

H3.3 p.G34W mutant-specific immunohistochemistry (IHC; clone RM263, commercially available) is a highly sensitive and specific surrogate marker of H3F3A p.G34W mutation in GCTB [56–58], being useful for practical diagnosis in primary [58] or recurrent, metastatic, and secondary malignant GCTB [59]. Although denosumab therapy may decrease p.G34W expression [22], evidence shows that spindle cells and cells in and around immature bone in denosumab-treated GCTBs are H3.3 p.G34W-positive by IHC, with H3F3A mutations consistently detected in corresponding samples [56, 58, 60, 61], which may predict relapse risk [55].

Although rare, malignant GCTB may occur, and studies suggest that p.G34W mutation is preserved [55]. One report, however, showed loss of one *H3F3A* allele (probably the mutant allele) in GCTB malignant component, leading to negative p.G34W IHC [62].

p63, a member of the p53 family of transcription factors, has also been studied as biomarker in GCTB diagnosis. p63 immunostaining has been used in diagnosis of head and neck squamous cell carcinoma, prostate adenocarcinoma (negative for p63 in opposition to p63-positive benign prostatic tissue) [63], and poorly differentiated squamous cell carcinoma [64]. p63 has also been shown to be highly expressed in GCTB mononuclear neoplastic cells [65–67], but its usefulness is still to be determined. A meta-analysis of eight different studies including 335 GCTB patients showed that p63 is a helpful marker for GCTB diagnosis in critically ill patients, although it cannot be recommended as a single definitive diagnostic marker [68].

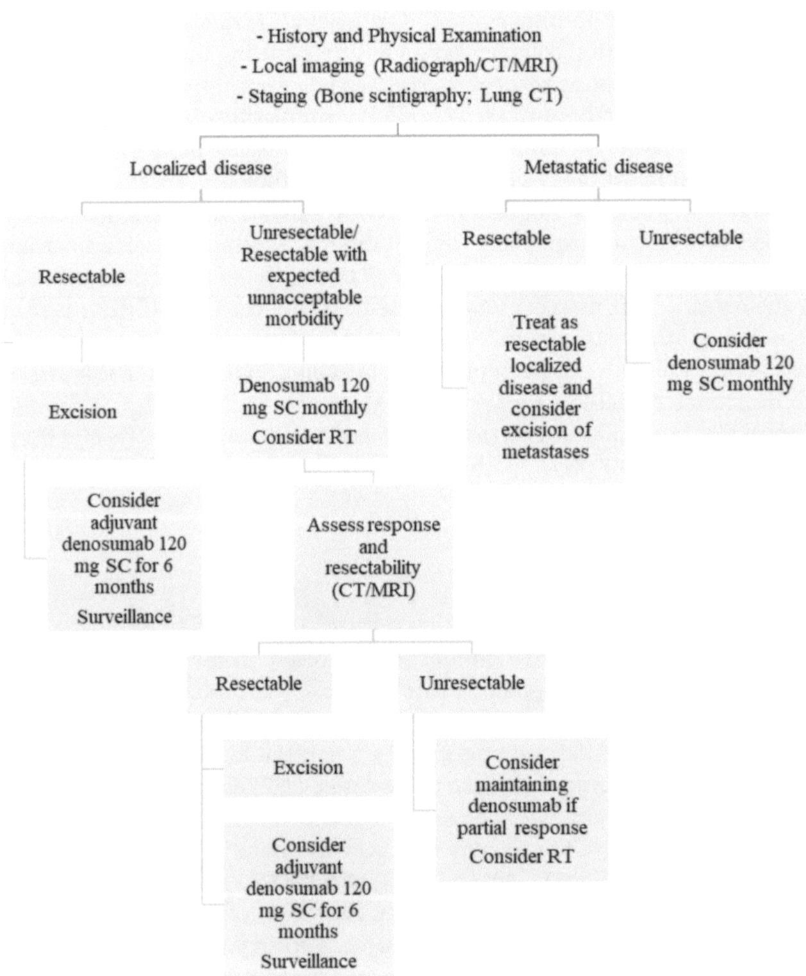

Figure 3.
Flowchart of GCTB treatment. Adapted from NCCN guidelines – Bone cancer [73]. CT, computorized tomography; MRI, magnetic resonance imaging; RT, radiation therapy; SC, subcutaneous.

Finally, it has been suggested that high RANKL, IL-6, TNFα, SDF-1, and MCP-1 expression may help predict GCTB metastatic potential and prognosis, warranting further studies [69].

3. Treatment overview

Treatment options for localized GCTB include *en bloc* resection or curettage with or without local adjuvants, like phenol, liquid nitrogen, or polymethylmethacrylate [70]. Radiation therapy (RT) can also be used as an alternative to surgery for local control, with 5-year local control rates of 80% [71]. However, RT is associated with risk of malignant transformation into high-grade sarcoma, making surgery the preferred option when possible. Contrarily to palliative care in irresectable or distant disease, systemic neoadjuvant or adjuvant therapy with the RANKL-binding fully human monoclonal antibody denosumab is still not established [70, 72]. A treatment algorithm is depicted in **Figure 3**.

4. Medical therapy

4.1 Denosumab

Denosumab is a fully human monoclonal antibody (IgG2) that binds with high affinity and specificity to RANKL [74], thereby inhibiting osteoclast-mediated osteolysis. Given GCTB pathophysiology and its association to RANKL/RANK pathway, denosumab has proven effective in this disease.

In patients with resectable GCTB, adjuvant denosumab at a 120 mg dosage administered subcutaneously every 28 days, with additional loading doses on days 8 and 15 on the first month, during 6 months after complete resection has been approved by both the Food and Drug Administration and European Medicines Agency [72, 75, 76]. However, this treatment is still debated. Studies supporting its use in the adjuvant setting are scarce and mostly rely in level IV evidence. Conversely, evidence from a systematic review by Luengo-Alonso [72] favored adjuvant denosumab, which showed a positive histological and clinical (pain relief) response. In patients with unresectable GCTB (either primary or recurrent) or when complete excision is possible but post-surgical severe morbidity and functional impairment is expected, neoadjuvant denosumab should be started (same dosing scheme as above) and response to treatment evaluated. Should the patient respond to denosumab and surgery be feasible with acceptable morbidity, then complete excision and possibly adjuvant denosumab for six months should be considered. On the other hand, the optimal denosumab duration is still debatable when treatment response is suboptimal or in cases of sacral or spinal GCTB, multiple lesions (including pulmonary metastases), or patient's clinical ineligibility for surgery. Denosumab should be considered until progression or unacceptable toxicity (e.g., osteonecrosis of the jaw), provided at least partial response is achieved.

4.2 Bisphosphonates

Bisphosphonates inhibit osteoclast-mediated bone resorption and are used in cancer patients, especially in bone metastases setting. In GCTB patients, denosumab is the preferred systemic treatment option. However, evidence regarding the use of adjuvant denosumab is not consistent and some studies show lack of benefit in local recurrence rates [77, 78]. Bisphosphonates, like zoledronic acid (ZA), can be an option in the adjuvant setting. A recent meta-analysis of case–control studies showed that the use of adjuvant bisphosphonates in patients submitted to intralesional curettage may decrease local recurrence rates, independently of Campanacci staging [79]. In patients undergoing wide resection, bisphosphonates seem to have no benefit in local recurrence. A phase II non-randomized clinical trial of adjuvant ZA after extensive curettage in GCTB patients showed that ZA failed to prevent local recurrence [80]. Another phase II multicentric, randomized, open-label clinical trial showed no benefit with adjuvant ZA, although the study was terminated earlier due to poor accrual [81]. The use of adjuvant bisphosphonates should be evaluated on a case-by-case basis. In unresectable or metastatic GCTB, clinical studies addressing the use of bisphosphonates are also scarce. Overall, the role of bisphosphonates in the treatment of patients with GCTB remains to be clearly defined.

4.3 Chemotherapy/systemic cytotoxic agents/interferon

Chemotherapy agents and interferon-α have also been used to treat GCTB, as reported in case reports and small series, but results were poor and there are no clinical trials to guide their use. Anecdotal small retrospective case series and case reports have documented the use of doxorubicin [82, 83], cyclophosphamide [84], cisplatin plus doxorubicin [85], combination therapy with vincristine, doxorubicin, cyclophosphamide and actinomycin-D, followed by high-dose methotrexate and vincristine [86], interferon alpha 2a [87] and interferon alpha 2b [88], with mixed results.

5. Conclusions and future directions

GCTB is a primary and mostly benign tumor of bone usually arising in the meta-epiphysis of long bones and more often affecting young patients. Despite its frequent benign nature, local recurrence rate is high and there is a non-negligible risk of distant metastization, namely to the lungs. Therefore, treatment should provide the best chance of curative outcome with minimal functional sequelae and quality of life impairment.

The main pillar of treatment is surgery, but systemic therapy has a role in adjuvant and palliative settings. Regarding GCTB pathophysiology, RANKL/RANK pathway is central to tumor development and denosumab, a monoclonal antibody against RANKL, is the most studied and most effective systemic therapy for the disease. Its use is particularly established in the palliative setting, i.e., in cases of unresectable disease, patient ineligibility for surgery, or lung involvement. Although less studied, bisphosphonates can also be an option. However, their role in GCTB medical management needs to be better clarified.

GCTB rare nature, particularly malignant GCTB, hampers the development of clinical trials to investigate new drugs for second-line treatment and establish the optimal treatment sequence (neo- vs. adjuvant denosumab or adjuvant denosumab vs. after recurrence, etc.). Currently, one clinical trial (NCT04255576) is studying the use of JMT103, a novel fully human IgG4 monoclonal antibody against RANKL, in GCTB [89]. Another clinical trial (NCT03449108) is using a different approach to address bone tumors, including GCTB [90], by studying the use of LN-145-S1, or autologous tumor infiltrating lymphocytes, in treatment-refractory or relapsed disease. As discussed above, mutations in cyclin D1, p53, and MET have been associated with GCTB malignant transformation and recurrence. This raises the hypothesis that cyclin-dependent kinase (CDK) inhibitors (e.g., ribociclib, palbociclib) and MET inhibitors (e.g., crizotinib) may be useful in this disease. Although these therapies have been approved in other tumors (CDK inhibitors in breast cancer and crizotinib in lung cancer), no studies are in place in GCTB yet. Another promising target is MMPs, specially MMP-2 and MMP-9, that play an important role in GCTB physiopathology, namely regarding tumor microenvironment, angiogenesis, invasion, and metastatic development. Preclinical studies in breast cancer used ML115, a bone-seeking MMP inhibitor, to prevent bone metastases [91], with promising results. Although still far from use in the clinical practice, this could be another potential therapy worth studying in GCTB. Several other clinical trials continue to investigate the use of denosumab, bisphosphonates, and local therapy (surgery/RT) [92–97].

Acknowledgements

We thank Joana Cavaco Silva for her contribution as a medical writer. Authors acknowledge Joana Cavaco Silva for manuscript revision.

Conflict of interest

The authors declare no conflict of interest.

Nomenclature

BMP-2	Bone morphogenetic protein 2
CCR2	C-C chemokine receptor type 2
CXCR4	C-X-C chemokine receptor type 4
C/EBPβ	CCAAT/enhancer binding protein beta
CT	Computorized tomography
CDK	Cyclin-kinase inhibitors
DC-STAMP	Dendritic cell-specific transmembrane protein
EMMPRIN	Extracellular matrix metalloproteinase inducer
FFPE	Formalin-Fixed Paraffin-Embedded
GCTB	Giant cell tumor of the bone
H3.3	Histone 3.3
IgG	Immunoglobulin G
IHC	Immunohistochemistry
IGF	Insulin-like growth factor
IL-1	Interleukin 1
M-CSF	Macrophage colony-stimulating factor
MIP-1α	Macrophage inflammatory protein 1-alpha;
MRI	Magnetic resonance imaging
MMP	Matrix metalloprotease
MCP-1	Monocyte chemoattractant protein-1
NFATc1	Nuclear factor of activated T cells c1
OC-STAMP	Osteoclast stimulatory transmembrane protein
PTHrP	Parathyroid hormone related peptide
RT	Radiation therapy
RANKL	Receptor activator of nuclear factor kappa-B ligand
RUNX2	Runt-related transcription factor 2
SC	Subcutaneous

SDF-1	Stromal cell-derived factor 1
TRAP	Tartrate-resistant acid phosphatase
TRAIL	TNF-related apoptosis inducing ligand
TGF-β	Transforming growth factor beta
TNF-α	Tumor necrosis factor-alpha
VEGF	Vascular endothelial growth factor
ZA	Zoledronic acid

Author details

Raquel Lopes-Brás[1*], Isabel Fernandes[1,2], Sandra Casimiro[2] and Luís Costa[1,2*]

1 Medical Oncology Department, Hospital de Santa Maria, Centro Hospitalar Universitário Lisboa Norte, Lisbon, Portugal

2 LCosta Lab, Instituto de Medicina Molecular – João Lobo Antunes, Faculdade de Medicina da Universidade de Lisboa, Lisbon, Portugal

*Address all correspondence to: raquellopesbras@gmail.com and luiscosta.oncology@gmail.com

References

[1] Athanasou NA, Bansal M, Forsyth R, Reid RP, Sapi Z. Giant cell tumour of bone. In: Fletcher C, Bridge J, Hogendoorn P, Mertens F, editors. WHO classification of tumours of soft tissue and bone. 4th ed. Lyon: International Agency for Research on Cancer (IARC); 2013. p. 321-4.

[2] Liede A, Bach BA, Stryker S, Hernandez RK, Sobocki P, Bennett B, et al. Regional variation and challenges in estimating the incidence of giant cell tumor of bone. The Journal of bone and joint surgery American volume. 2014;96 (23):1999-2007.

[3] Larsson SE, Lorentzon R, Boquist L. Giant-cell tumor of bone. A demographic, clinical, and histopathological study of all cases recorded in the Swedish Cancer Registry for the years 1958 through 1968. The Journal of bone and joint surgery American volume. 1975;57(2):167-173.

[4] Goldenberg RR, Campbell CJ, Bonfiglio M. Giant-cell tumor of bone. An analysis of two hundred and eighteen cases. The Journal of bone and joint surgery American volume. 1970;52 (4):619-664.

[5] Amanatullah DF, Clark TR, Lopez MJ, Borys D, Tamurian RM. Giant cell tumor of bone. Orthopedics. 2014;37(2):112-120.

[6] Chan CM, Adler Z, Reith JD, Gibbs CP, Jr. Risk factors for pulmonary metastases from giant cell tumor of bone. The Journal of bone and joint surgery American volume. 2015;97(5):420-428.

[7] Enneking WF. A system of staging musculoskeletal neoplasms. Clinical orthopaedics and related research. 1986 (204):9-24.

[8] Siebenrock KA, Unni KK, Rock MG. Giant-cell tumour of bone metastasising to the lungs. A long-term follow-up. The Journal of bone and joint surgery British volume. 1998;80(1):43-47.

[9] Rock MG, Pritchard DJ, Unni KK. Metastases from histologically benign giant-cell tumor of bone. The Journal of bone and joint surgery American volume. 1984;66(2):269-274.

[10] Gong L, Liu W, Sun X, Sajdik C, Tian X, Niu X, et al. Histological and clinical characteristics of malignant giant cell tumor of bone. Virchows Archiv: an international journal of pathology. 2012;460(3):327-334.

[11] Hoch B, Inwards C, Sundaram M, Rosenberg AE. Multicentric giant cell tumor of bone. Clinicopathologic analysis of thirty cases. The Journal of bone and joint surgery American volume. 2006;88(9):1998-2008.

[12] Sobti A, Agrawal P, Agarwala S, Agarwal M. Giant Cell Tumor of Bone - An Overview. Arch Bone Jt Surg. 2016;4 (1):2-9.

[13] Campanacci M, Baldini N, Boriani S, Sudanese A. Giant-cell tumor of bone. JBJS. 1987;69(1).

[14] Jaffe HL. Giant cell tumor of bone: Its pathologic appearance, grading, supposed variants and treatment. Arch Pathol. 1940;30:993-1031.

[15] Palmerini E, Picci P, Reichardt P, Downey G. Malignancy in Giant Cell Tumor of Bone: A Review of the Literature. Technology in cancer research & treatment. 2019;18: 1533033819840000.

[16] Hu P, Zhao L, Zhang H, Yu X, Wang Z, Ye Z, et al. Recurrence Rates and Risk Factors for Primary Giant Cell Tumors around the Knee: A Multicentre Retrospective Study in China. Scientific reports. 2016;6:36332.

[17] Lipplaa A, Dijkstra S, Gelderblom H. Challenges of denosumab in giant cell tumor of bone, and other giant cell-rich tumors of bone. Current opinion in oncology. 2019;31(4):329-335.

[18] Tubbs WS, Brown LR, Beabout JW, Rock MG, Unni KK. Benign giant-cell tumor of bone with pulmonary metastases: clinical findings and radiologic appearance of metastases in 13 cases. AJR American journal of roentgenology. 1992;158(2):331-334.

[19] Beebe-Dimmer JL, Cetin K, Fryzek JP, Schuetze SM, Schwartz K. The epidemiology of malignant giant cell tumors of bone: an analysis of data from the Surveillance, Epidemiology and End Results Program (1975-2004). Rare Tumors. 2009;1(2):e52-e.

[20] Rock MG, Sim FH, Unni KK, Witrak GA, Frassica FJ, Schray MF, et al. Secondary malignant giant-cell tumor of bone. Clinicopathological assessment of nineteen patients. The Journal of bone and joint surgery American volume. 1986;68(7):1073-1079.

[21] Kuhn J, Sapra A. Osteoclastoma. StatPearls. Treasure Island (FL)2020.

[22] Noh BJ, Park YK. Giant cell tumor of bone: updated molecular pathogenesis and tumor biology. Human pathology. 2018;81:1-8.

[23] Branstetter DG, Nelson SD, Manivel JC, Blay JY, Chawla S, Thomas DM, et al. Denosumab induces tumor reduction and bone formation in patients with giant-cell tumor of bone. Clinical cancer research: an official journal of the American Association for Cancer Research. 2012;18(16):4415-4424.

[24] Maggiani F, Forsyth R, Hogendoorn PC, Krenacs T, Athanasou NA. The immunophenotype of osteoclasts and macrophage polykaryons. J Clin Pathol. 2011;64(8): 701-705.

[25] Doussis IA, Puddle B, Athanasou NA. Immunophenotype of multinucleated and mononuclear cells in giant cell lesions of bone and soft tissue. J Clin Pathol. 1992;45(5):398-404.

[26] Atkins GJ, Haynes DR, Graves SE, Evdokiou A, Hay S, Bouralexis S, et al. Expression of osteoclast differentiation signals by stromal elements of giant cell tumors. Journal of bone and mineral research: the official journal of the American Society for Bone and Mineral Research. 2000;15(4):640-649.

[27] Forsyth RG, De Boeck G, Baelde JJ, Taminiau AH, Uyttendaele D, Roels H, et al. CD33+ CD14- phenotype is characteristic of multinuclear osteoclast-like cells in giant cell tumor of bone. Journal of bone and mineral research: the official journal of the American Society for Bone and Mineral Research. 2009;24(1):70-77.

[28] Goldring SR, Roelke MS, Petrison KK, Bhan AK. Human giant cell tumors of bone identification and characterization of cell types. J Clin Invest. 1987;79(2):483-491.

[29] Lau YS, Sabokbar A, Gibbons CL, Giele H, Athanasou N. Phenotypic and molecular studies of giant-cell tumors of bone and soft tissue. Human pathology. 2005;36(9):945-954.

[30] Behjati S, Tarpey PS, Presneau N, Scheipl S, Pillay N, Van Loo P, et al. Distinct H3F3A and H3F3B driver mutations define chondroblastoma and giant cell tumor of bone. Nat Genet. 2013;45(12):1479-1482.

[31] Wulling M, Delling G, Kaiser E. The origin of the neoplastic stromal cell in giant cell tumor of bone. Human pathology. 2003;34(10):983-993.

[32] Huang L, Teng XY, Cheng YY, Lee KM, Kumta SM. Expression of preosteoblast markers and Cbfa-1 and Osterix gene transcripts in stromal

tumour cells of giant cell tumour of bone. Bone. 2004;34(3):393-401.

[33] Murata A, Fujita T, Kawahara N, Tsuchiya H, Tomita K. Osteoblast lineage properties in giant cell tumors of bone. J Orthop Sci. 2005;10(6):581-588.

[34] Singh S, Mak IW, Cowan RW, Turcotte R, Singh G, Ghert M. The role of TWIST as a regulator in giant cell tumor of bone. J Cell Biochem. 2011;112(9):2287-2295.

[35] Gorunova L, Vult von Steyern F, Storlazzi CT, Bjerkehagen B, Folleras G, Heim S, et al. Cytogenetic analysis of 101 giant cell tumors of bone: nonrandom patterns of telomeric associations and other structural aberrations. Genes Chromosomes Cancer. 2009;48(7):583-602.

[36] Horvai AE, Kramer MJ, Garcia JJ, O'Donnell RJ. Distribution and prognostic significance of human telomerase reverse transcriptase (hTERT) expression in giant-cell tumor of bone. Mod Pathol. 2008;21(4):423-430.

[37] Schwartz HS, Butler MG, Jenkins RB, Miller DA, Moses HL. Telomeric associations and consistent growth factor overexpression detected in giant cell tumor of bone. Cancer Genet Cytogenet. 1991;56(2):263-276.

[38] Schwartz HS, Eskew JD, Butler MG. Clonality studies in giant cell tumor of bone. J Orthop Res. 2002;20(2):387-390.

[39] Matsubayashi S, Nakashima M, Kumagai K, Egashira M, Naruke Y, Kondo H, et al. Immunohistochemical analyses of beta-catenin and cyclin D1 expression in giant cell tumor of bone (GCTB): a possible role of Wnt pathway in GCTB tumorigenesis. Pathol Res Pract. 2009;205(9):626-633.

[40] Wang T, Jiao J, Zhang H, Zhou W, Li Z, Han S, et al. TGF-beta induced PAR-1 expression promotes tumor progression and osteoclast differentiation in giant cell tumor of bone. Int J Cancer. 2017;141(8):1630-1642.

[41] Joyner CJ, Quinn JM, Triffitt JT, Owen ME, Athanasou NA. Phenotypic characterisation of mononuclear and multinucleated cells of giant cell tumour of bone. Bone Miner. 1992;16(1):37-48.

[42] Miyamoto N, Higuchi Y, Tajima M, Ito M, Tsurudome M, Nishio M, et al. Spindle-shaped cells derived from giant-cell tumor of bone support differentiation of blood monocytes to osteoclast-like cells. J Orthop Res. 2000;18(4):647-654.

[43] Roux S, Quinn J, Pichaud F, Orcel P, Chastre E, Jullienne A, et al. Human cord blood monocytes undergo terminal osteoclast differentiation in vitro in the presence of culture medium conditioned by giant cell tumor of bone. J Cell Physiol. 1996;168(3):489-498.

[44] Atkins GJ, Bouralexis S, Haynes DR, Graves SE, Geary SM, Evdokiou A, et al. Osteoprotegerin inhibits osteoclast formation and bone resorbing activity in giant cell tumors of bone. Bone. 2001;28(4):370-377.

[45] Zheng MH, Fan Y, Smith A, Wysocki S, Papadimitriou JM, Wood DJ. Gene expression of monocyte chemoattractant protein-1 in giant cell tumors of bone osteoclastoma: possible involvement in CD68+ macrophage-like cell migration. J Cell Biochem. 1998;70(1):121-129.

[46] Yu Q, Stamenkovic I. Cell surface-localized matrix metalloproteinase-9 proteolytically activates TGF-beta and promotes tumor invasion and angiogenesis. Genes Dev. 2000;14(2):163-176.

[47] Liao TS, Yurgelun MB, Chang SS, Zhang HZ, Murakami K, Blaine TA,

et al. Recruitment of osteoclast precursors by stromal cell derived factor-1 (SDF-1) in giant cell tumor of bone. J Orthop Res. 2005;23(1):203-209.

[48] Ng PK, Tsui SK, Lau CP, Wong CH, Wong WH, Huang L, et al. CCAAT/enhancer binding protein beta is up-regulated in giant cell tumor of bone and regulates RANKL expression. J Cell Biochem. 2010;110(2):438-446.

[49] Mak IW, Turcotte RE, Ghert M. Parathyroid hormone-related protein (PTHrP) modulates adhesion, migration and invasion in bone tumor cells. Bone. 2013;55(1):198-207.

[50] Miyamoto H, Suzuki T, Miyauchi Y, Iwasaki R, Kobayashi T, Sato Y, et al. Osteoclast stimulatory transmembrane protein and dendritic cell-specific transmembrane protein cooperatively modulate cell-cell fusion to form osteoclasts and foreign body giant cells. Journal of bone and mineral research: the official journal of the American Society for Bone and Mineral Research. 2012;27(6):1289-1297.

[51] Hemingway F, Taylor R, Knowles HJ, Athanasou NA. RANKL-independent human osteoclast formation with APRIL, BAFF, NGF, IGF I and IGF II. Bone. 2011;48 (4):938-944.

[52] Gohda J, Akiyama T, Koga T, Takayanagi H, Tanaka S, Inoue J. RANK-mediated amplification of TRAF6 signaling leads to NFATc1 induction during osteoclastogenesis. EMBO J. 2005;24(4):790-799.

[53] Pilkington MF, Sims SM, Dixon SJ. Transforming growth factor-beta induces osteoclast ruffling and chemotaxis: potential role in osteoclast recruitment. Journal of bone and mineral research: the official journal of the American Society for Bone and Mineral Research. 2001;16(7): 1237-1247.

[54] Si AI, Huang L, Xu J, Kumta SM, Wood D, Zheng MH. Expression and localization of extracellular matrix metalloproteinase inducer in giant cell tumor of bone. J Cell Biochem. 2003;89 (6):1154-1163.

[55] Yamamoto H, Ishihara S, Toda Y, Oda Y. Histone H3.3 mutation in giant cell tumor of bone: an update in pathology. Med Mol Morphol. 2020;53 (1):1-6.

[56] Yamamoto H, Iwasaki T, Yamada Y, Matsumoto Y, Otsuka H, Yoshimoto M, et al. Diagnostic utility of histone H3.3 G34W, G34R, and G34V mutant-specific antibodies for giant cell tumors of bone. Human pathology. 2018;73: 41-50.

[57] Amary F, Berisha F, Ye H, Gupta M, Gutteridge A, Baumhoer D, et al. H3F3A (Histone 3.3) G34W Immunohistochemistry: A Reliable Marker Defining Benign and Malignant Giant Cell Tumor of Bone. Am J Surg Pathol. 2017;41(8):1059-1068.

[58] Luke J, von Baer A, Schreiber J, Lubbehusen C, Breining T, Mellert K, et al. H3F3A mutation in giant cell tumour of the bone is detected by immunohistochemistry using a monoclonal antibody against the G34W mutated site of the histone H3.3 variant. Histopathology. 2017;71(1):125-133.

[59] Tsukamoto Y, Futani H, Kihara T, Watanabe T, Kumanishi S, Matsuo S, et al. An extremely rare case of primary malignancy in giant cell tumor of bone, arising in the right femur and harboring H3F3A mutation. Pathol Res Pract. 2018;214(9):1504-1509.

[60] Kato I, Furuya M, Matsuo K, Kawabata Y, Tanaka R, Ohashi K. Giant cell tumours of bone treated with denosumab: histological, immunohistochemical and H3F3A mutation analyses. Histopathology. 2018;72(6):914-922.

[61] Girolami I, Mancini I, Simoni A, Baldi GG, Simi L, Campanacci D, et al. Denosumab treated giant cell tumour of bone: a morphological, immunohistochemical and molecular analysis of a series. J Clin Pathol. 2016; 69(3):240-247.

[62] Yoshida KI, Nakano Y, Honda-Kitahara M, Wakai S, Motoi T, Ogura K, et al. Absence of H3F3A mutation in a subset of malignant giant cell tumor of bone. Mod Pathol. 2019;32(12): 1751-1761.

[63] Shiran MS, Tan GC, Sabariah AR, Rampal L, Phang KS. p63 as a complimentary basal cell specific marker to high molecular weight-cytokeratin in distinguishing prostatic carcinoma from benign prostatic lesions. Med J Malaysia. 2007;62(1):36-39.

[64] Zhang H, Liu J, Cagle PT, Allen TC, Laga AC, Zander DS. Distinction of pulmonary small cell carcinoma from poorly differentiated squamous cell carcinoma: an immunohistochemical approach. Mod Pathol. 2005;18(1): 111-118.

[65] Shooshtarizadeh T, Rahimi M, Movahedinia S. P63 expression as a biomarker discriminating giant cell tumor of bone from other giant cell-rich bone lesions. Pathol Res Pract. 2016;212 (10):876-879.

[66] Yanagisawa M, Kakizaki H, Okada K, Torigoe T, Kusumi T. p63 as a prognostic marker for giant cell tumor of bone. Ups J Med Sci. 2013;118(1): 23-28.

[67] Lee CH, Espinosa I, Jensen KC, Subramanian S, Zhu SX, Varma S, et al. Gene expression profiling identifies p63 as a diagnostic marker for giant cell tumor of the bone. Mod Pathol. 2008;21 (5):531-539.

[68] Wan Z, Lee CW, Yuan S, Lee OK. Can p63 serve as a biomarker for diagnosing giant cell tumor of bone? A systematic review and meta-analysis. Sao Paulo Med J. 2020;138(5):393-399.

[69] Muheremu A, Niu X. Pulmonary metastasis of giant cell tumor of bones. World J Surg Oncol. 2014;12:261.

[70] Casali PG, Bielack S, Abecassis N, Aro HT, Bauer S, Biagini R, et al. Bone sarcomas: ESMO-PaedCan-EURACAN Clinical Practice Guidelines for diagnosis, treatment and follow-up. Annals of Oncology. 2018;29:iv79-iv95.

[71] Shi W, Indelicato DJ, Reith J, Smith KB, Morris CG, Scarborough MT, et al. Radiotherapy in the management of giant cell tumor of bone. American journal of clinical oncology. 2013;36(5): 505-508.

[72] Luengo-Alonso G, Mellado-Romero M, Shemesh S, Ramos-Pascua L, Pretell-Mazzini J. Denosumab treatment for giant-cell tumor of bone: a systematic review of the literature. Archives of orthopaedic and trauma surgery. 2019; 139(10):1339-1349.

[73] National Comprehensive Cancer Network (NCCN). Bone Cancer (Version 1.2021) 2021 [Available from: https://www.nccn.org/professionals/physician_gls/pdf/bone.pdf.

[74] Bekker PJ, Holloway DL, Rasmussen AS, Murphy R, Martin SW, Leese PT, et al. A single-dose placebo-controlled study of AMG 162, a fully human monoclonal antibody to RANKL, in postmenopausal women. Journal of bone and mineral research: the official journal of the American Society for Bone and Mineral Research. 2004;19(7): 1059-1066.

[75] Chawla S, Henshaw R, Seeger L, Choy E, Blay JY, Ferrari S, et al. Safety and efficacy of denosumab for adults and skeletally mature adolescents with giant cell tumour of bone: interim analysis of an open-label, parallel-

group, phase 2 study. The Lancet Oncology. 2013;14(9):901-908.

[76] Xgeva - Summary of Product Characteristics: European Medicines Agency; 2011 [updated 2016. Available from: https://www.ema.europa.eu/en/documents/product-information/xgeva-epar-product-information_en.pdf.

[77] Müller DA, Beltrami G, Scoccianti G, Campanacci DA, Franchi A, Capanna R. Risks and benefits of combining denosumab and surgery in giant cell tumor of bone-a case series. World J Surg Oncol. 2016;14 (1):281.

[78] Errani C, Tsukamoto S, Leone G, Righi A, Akahane M, Tanaka Y, et al. Denosumab May Increase the Risk of Local Recurrence in Patients with Giant-Cell Tumor of Bone Treated with Curettage. The Journal of bone and joint surgery American volume. 2018;100(6): 496-504.

[79] Shi M, Chen L, Wang Y, Wang W, Zhang Y, Yan S. Effect of bisphosphonates on local recurrence of giant cell tumor of bone: a meta-analysis. Cancer Manag Res. 2019;11: 669-680.

[80] Gouin F, Rochwerger AR, Di Marco A, Rosset P, Bonnevialle P, Fiorenza F, et al. Adjuvant treatment with zoledronic acid after extensive curettage for giant cell tumours of bone. European Journal of Cancer. 2014;50 (14):2425-2431.

[81] Lipplaa A, Kroep JR, van der Heijden L, Jutte PC, Hogendoorn PCW, Dijkstra S, et al. Adjuvant Zoledronic Acid in High-Risk Giant Cell Tumor of Bone: A Multicenter Randomized Phase II Trial. The oncologist. 2019;24(7):889-e421.

[82] Dominkus M, Ruggieri P, Bertoni F, Briccoli A, Picci P, Rocca M, et al. Histologically verified lung metastases in benign giant cell tumours–14 cases from a single institution. Int Orthop. 2006;30(6):499-504.

[83] Yamamoto M, Fukushima T, Sakamoto S, Tomonaga M. Giant cell tumor of the sphenoid bone: long-term follow-up of two cases after chemotherapy. Surgical neurology. 1998;49(5):547-552.

[84] Osaka S, Toriyama M, Taira K, Sano S, Saotome K. Analysis of giant cell tumor of bone with pulmonary metastases. Clinical orthopaedics and related research. 1997(335):253-261.

[85] Stewart DJ, Belanger R, Benjamin RS. Prolonged disease-free survival following surgical debulking and high-dose cisplatin/doxorubicin in a patient with bulky metastases from giant cell tumor of bone refractory to "standard" chemotherapy. American journal of clinical oncology. 1995;18(2): 144-148.

[86] Mella O, Dahl O, Bang G, Engedal H, Gøthlin J, Lunde OD. Chemotherapy of a malignant, metastasizing giant-cell tumor of bone: report of an unusual case and the response to combination chemotherapy. Cancer. 1982;50(2):207-211.

[87] Kaiser U, Neumann K, Havemann K. Generalised giant-cell tumour of bone: successful treatment of pulmonary metastases with interferon alpha, a case report. Journal of cancer research and clinical oncology. 1993;119 (5):301-303.

[88] Wei F, Liu X, Liu Z, Jiang L, Dang G, Ma Q, et al. Interferon alfa-2b for recurrent and metastatic giant cell tumor of the spine: report of two cases. Spine. 2010;35(24):E1418-E1422.

[89] Efficacy and Safety of JMT103 in Patients With Giant Cell Tumor of Bone.

[90] LN-145 or LN-145-S1 in Treating Patients With Relapsed or Refractory

Ovarian Cancer, Anaplastic Thyroid Cancer, Osteosarcoma, or Other Bone and Soft Tissue Sarcomas.

[91] Tauro M, Lynch CC. Bone seeking matrix metalloproteinase-2 (MMP-2) inhibitors can prevent bone metastatic breast cancer. Annals of Oncology. 2019;30:iii60-iii1.

[92] Long-term Safety Follow-up of Subjects With Giant Cell Tumor of Bone Treated With Denosumab in Study 20062004.

[93] Safety and Efficacy of Post-operative Denosumab Strategy for Giant Cell Tumor of Bone Treatment in China.

[94] Study of XGEVA® (Denosumab) in Chinese Adults and Skeletally Mature Adolescents With Giant Cell Tumor of the Bone.

[95] Safety and Efficacy Study of Denosumab in Patients With Recurrent or Unresectable Giant Cell Tumor of Bone.

[96] Local Bisphosphonate Effect on Recurrence Rate in Extremity Giant Cell Tumor of Bone.

[97] Giant Cell Tumor of the Extremities Treated With Surgery and/or Medical Treatment.

Chapter 4

Osteosarcoma

Gottardo Bianchi, Leticia Gaiero, Nicolas Casales, Claudio Silveri and Ana C. Belzarena

Abstract

Osteogenic sarcoma is the most common primary bone cancer frequently affecting children and teenagers. Despite many years of research, little have the survival rates changed in the last fifty years. Early diagnosis, a complete systemic treatment program with a good tumor response and adequate margins continue to be the main determinants of patients' prognosis in this disease. Neoadjuvant chemotherapy followed by surgery and subsequent adjuvant systemic treatment remain the standard of care. Numerous reconstruction options available provide these patients better function and improved quality of life.

Keywords: osteosarcoma, bone primary malignant tumor, osteogenic sarcoma

1. Introduction

Osteosarcoma, also known as osteogenic sarcoma, is a primary bone malignancy characterized for the production of osteoid, the mineralized portion of bone matrix [1]. Different from what its name suggests the origin of the tumor is not bone itself, but mesenchymal stem cells and osteosarcomas can also be found in soft tissues unrelated to any bone [2]. The incidence is approximately 1000 new cases each year in the United States [3]. Osteosarcoma is the third most common cancer in adolescents and is the most frequent primary bone malignant tumor in this age group. The peak incidence is between the second and third decade of life, although there is a second peak of patients aged older than 60 years of age [4, 5]. This tumor can subclassified according to histologic grade, location within the bone and the histologic characteristics of the matrix, more than 90% are of high grade, intramedullary location conventional ones [6]. The most common histologic subtypes are osteoblastic, chondroblastic, fibroblastic and telangiectatic. Additionally, these tumors can be classified as primary or secondary, depending on if the origin is in normal bone or altered bone due to prior pathology, for example Paget's disease, or radiation [7]. From a genetic perspective, osteosarcomas are characterized by highly disorganized genomic aberrations rather than a constant genetic alteration commonly found in other tumors [8]. Despite this, it has been linked to alterations in some specific genetic pathways expressed as syndromes. Such as Li-Fraumeni syndrome or Rothmund-Thomson syndrome or an alteration of the Rb protein causing retinoblastoma early in life as well as osteogenic sarcomas [9].

IntechOpen

2. Clinical presentation

Osteosarcomas most commonly occur in the metaphysis of long bones, for the most part around the knee in the distal femur (43%0 or proximal tibia (23%), followed in frequency by the humerus (10%) (**Figure 1**) [10]. One in ten patients has a tumor of axial location, most commonly in the pelvis. Tumors of axial location tend to have a worse prognosis with higher recurrence rates and more advanced stages at presentation [10–12]. Patients complaint about intermittent pain and swelling, the pain is known to be severe enough to awake the patient during sleep hours [13]. Pain of a high intensity can potentially be an indication of an impending pathological fracture, fact that occurs in up to 10% of these patients [14]. A pathological fracture may represent a more aggressive tumor and the microRNA profile of tumors that fractured have been shown to be different that those without a break. Additionally, tumors that presented with a fracture were associated with a higher risk of metastatic spread as well as a worse prognosis overall [14].

About 20% of osteosarcoma patients have metastatic disease at presentation. Most of those secondary lesions are in the lung, bone being the second most common spread location [10]. Tumor size has been implicated as a risk factor for lung spread [15]. When osteogenic sarcoma presents in older population, there is a more frequent axial location compared to younger patients, being almost 40% of the elderly patients versus 10% in children and teenagers [16]. Additionally, the older patients tend to have larger tumors, more frequency of metastatic disease at presentation and a worse general prognosis with less opportunity for limb salvage procedures and inability to receive the full systemic treatment protocol as compared to younger patients [17]. Moreover, when the chemotherapy response seems to

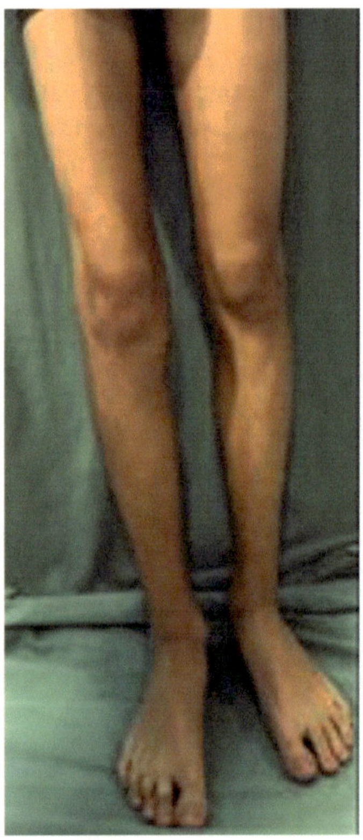

Figure 1.
Fifteen-year-old patient with a left proximal tibia osteosarcoma, presented with local pain and swelling.

be poorer in these patients with a lower percentage of necrosis noted on the post-chemotherapy tumor resection piece [10]. The 5-year overall survival is 50% for the elderly when surgical treatment is feasible, when surgery is not an option that rate drops to 8% [18].

3. Staging

The assessment of osteosarcoma patients usually begins with orthogonal plain radiographs of the site of pain or mass. Plain films usually reveal an aggressive appearing lesion that prompts more advanced imaging studies such as a CT scan or ideally an MRI with and without contrast of the entire affected bone. On radiographic imaging the lesions may be more blastic, lytic or mixed pattern depending on the osteosarcoma subtype. In more advanced cases, there will be cortical permeation and an associated soft tissue component, although this is a more common finding in Ewing's sarcomas [19]. For purely lytic lesions, radiographic evidence is only present when a substantial percentage of the bone has been affected (30–50%), thus the recommendation in cases of persistent symptoms is to proceed with an MRI even with a negative plain film [20]. Additional findings on radiographs include a wide area of transition, cortical destruction and a periosteal reaction such as Codman's triangle or a sunburnt pattern (**Figure 2**) [21].

The next imaging study should be a full bone length MRI with and without contrast of the affected area, this will serve diagnostic and staging purposes as well, since it has the ability of detecting skip lesions. MRI studies provide information regarding the complete extent of the tumor within the bone, and its closeness to surrounding structures such as vessels and nerves. Additionally, it provides information regarding joint invasion, and, extremely important in the pediatric population, physis involvement by the tumor [22]. This information will dictate the proposed surgical intervention (**Figure 3**). After neoadjuvant chemotherapy and prior to the definitive surgical treatment a new MRI with and without contrast of the affected bone must be obtained for tumor re-assessment.

Following the initial images, usually proceeds a close or open biopsy of the lesion for pathology confirmation of the diagnosis and grading of the tumor. It is

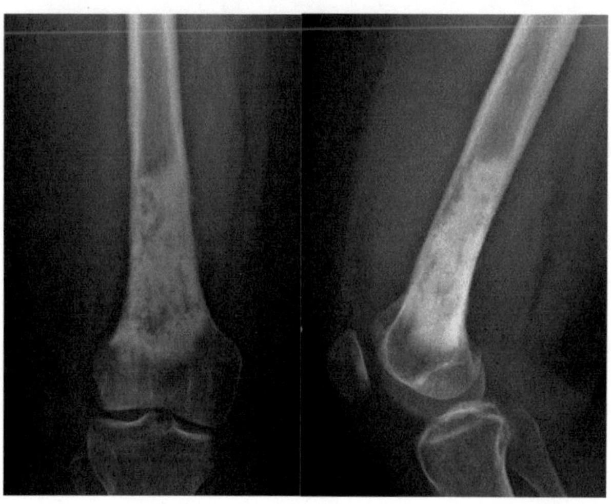

Figure 2.
Radiographic images of a patient with a distal femur conventional, central, osteoblastic, high grade osteosarcoma. The tumor presents a mixed, blastic and lytic, moth-eaten pattern.

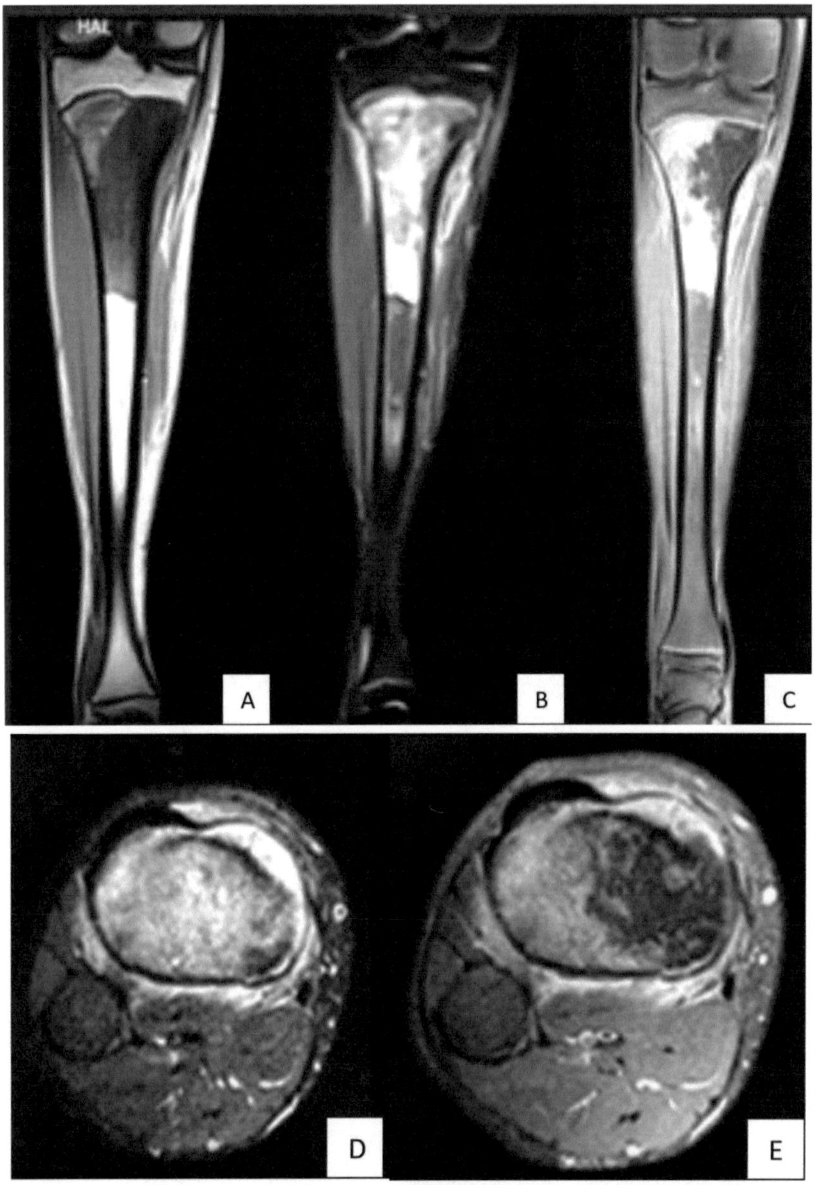

Figure 3.
MRI of the tibia of a 15-year-old patient with an osteoblastic osteosarcoma of the proximal tibia respecting the physis (D, E). T1-weighted sequence (A), stir sequence (B) and T1-fat suppressed post contrast sequence (C).

paramount that the biopsy is performed by a surgeon specialized and with experience in bone tumors, so that it can be done following important principles inherent to the specialty and have those not be respected it can potentially hinder the possibility of a limb salvage procedure for the patient [23].

Once the diagnosis of osteosarcoma has been confirmed, the next step is to proceed with staging of the patient. Approximately, 20% of patients debut with stage IV cancer [24]. Osteosarcomas are known to spread most commonly to lungs, 80% of the metastases, followed by bones (10%) [25, 26]. Therefore, the next imaging studies will be directed to assess the most common sites of spread. The lung assessment is performed with a non-contrasted chest CT and the bone staging can be performed by a bone scan or, more recently, with a PET-CT scan (**Figures 4** and **5**).

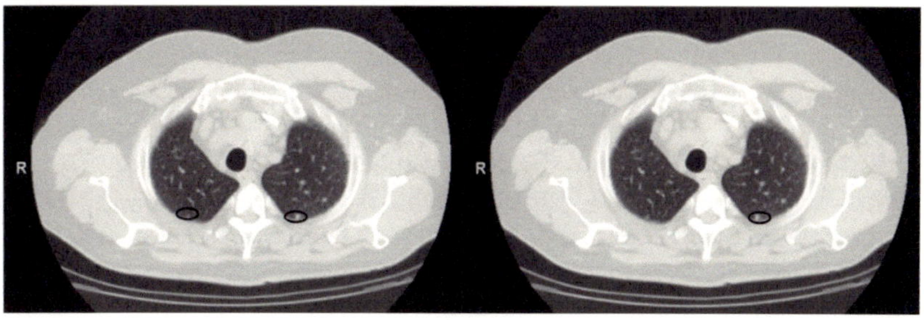

Figure 4.
Non-contrasted chest CT depicting peripheral lung nodules (circled) consistent with metastatic osteosarcoma.

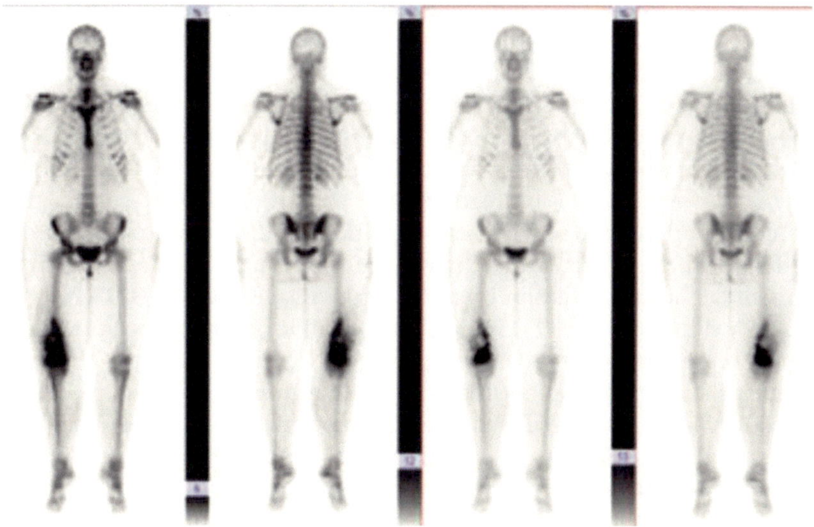

Figure 5.
Tecnecium-99 bone scan of a patient with a distal femur osteosarcoma. No other bone lesions were present.

Patients with metastatic disease at presentation have a worse prognosis than those with localized disease having an overall survival at 5 years of 40% or less [27]. Bone metastases have a particularly worse prognosis with higher rates of local recurrences and an overall survival of 13% [26].

Additional studies prior to the start of treatment, will be oriented at making a basal assessment of organs potentially affected by chemotherapy. Consequently, the patient will obtain an echocardiogram, kidney function studies, hemogram and complete metabolic panel as well as an audiology test [13]. Additionally, patients should be referred for fertility counseling since the systemic treatment is known to decrease the chances of conceiving even many years after the finalization of chemotherapy. Male patients present with particularly worse chances of conceiving than females and the cumulative dose of the drugs used seem to be the most important determinant factor to predict the ability to conceive after treatment [28].

4. Treatment

Currently, the treatment of localized osteogenic sarcoma is the same, independent of subtype and despite its different behaviors and genetic profiles, and includes a plan of neoadjuvant chemotherapy, followed by local treatment with surgical resection with a subsequent round of adjuvant chemotherapy [29]. This plan was first implemented in the 1970's and improved long-term survival rates from its original 20% to the current 70%, which has remained unchanged for the past five decades [30]. The three main reasons for treatment failure are local recurrences, distant disease spread and the development of drug resistance [31].

Systemic treatment for young patients includes two cycles of 5 weeks with high dose methotrexate, doxorubicin and cisplatin (MAP) [32]. Once the neoadjuvant cycle has finalized new imaging studies are obtained and the surgical procedure is planned. The resection piece is afterwards analyzed by the pathologist who must inform the percentage of necrosis, a key factor of prognostic significance and a proxy for the tumor chemotherapy response [33]. Following local treatment, 3 to 6 cycles of the same drug regimen (MAP) are given to the patient.

Before the implementation of chemotherapy as part of the treatment plan of these patients, even the ones with localized disease, most patients underwent a limb amputation, and despite this aggressive procedure still had poor survival rates. Nowadays, the standard of care for most patients is a limb salvage procedure which has shown similar survival rates to an amputation when systemic treatment was added with a much-improved function and quality of life [34, 35]. The main goal of limb salvage procedures is to completely resect the tumor while preserving important structures for the limb survival as well as the patient's function. Several studies have addressed the importance of achieving adequate margins in a resection as a determinant factor for the feasibility of the limb salvage option [33, 36, 37]. Local recurrences, which occur in 10–15% of these patients, has been linked to the margin adequacy as a predicting factor [38].

Once a decision has been made regarding the limb salvage procedure, several options present in terms of reconstruction alternatives, all with their specific advantages and disadvantages. Resection and reconstruction with an endoprosthetic device, a non-biologic option, is the main trend worldwide currently (**Figure 6**). While the biologic alternatives include allografts, vascularized fibula, distraction osteogenesis or recycled and sterilized bone autograft [39–43]. The latter can be achieved through several different techniques such as pasteurization, irradiation, autoclave or most recently the use of liquid nitrogen [44].

Endoprosthetic reconstructions have shown good results in terms of function at short and medium-term. Among its disadvantages it is its high cost, low accessibility in some countries and limited survival (50–76% at 10 years) with a high rate of

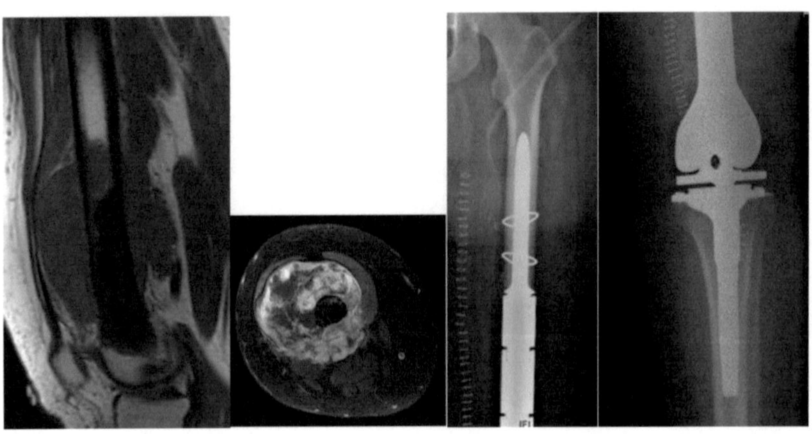

Figure 6.
Distal femur osteogenic sarcoma resection and reconstruction with a distal femur endoprosthetic device non-cemented.

reoperation specially in pediatric patients, an age where primary bone malignant tumors are most frequent [45]. Allografts require a bone bank with matching bone pieces. Furthermore, allografts have the potential to transmit diseases and, in some cases, patient acceptance may be an added obstacle [46]. Bone transport is a lengthy complex treatment with multiple surgical procedures usually involved [43].

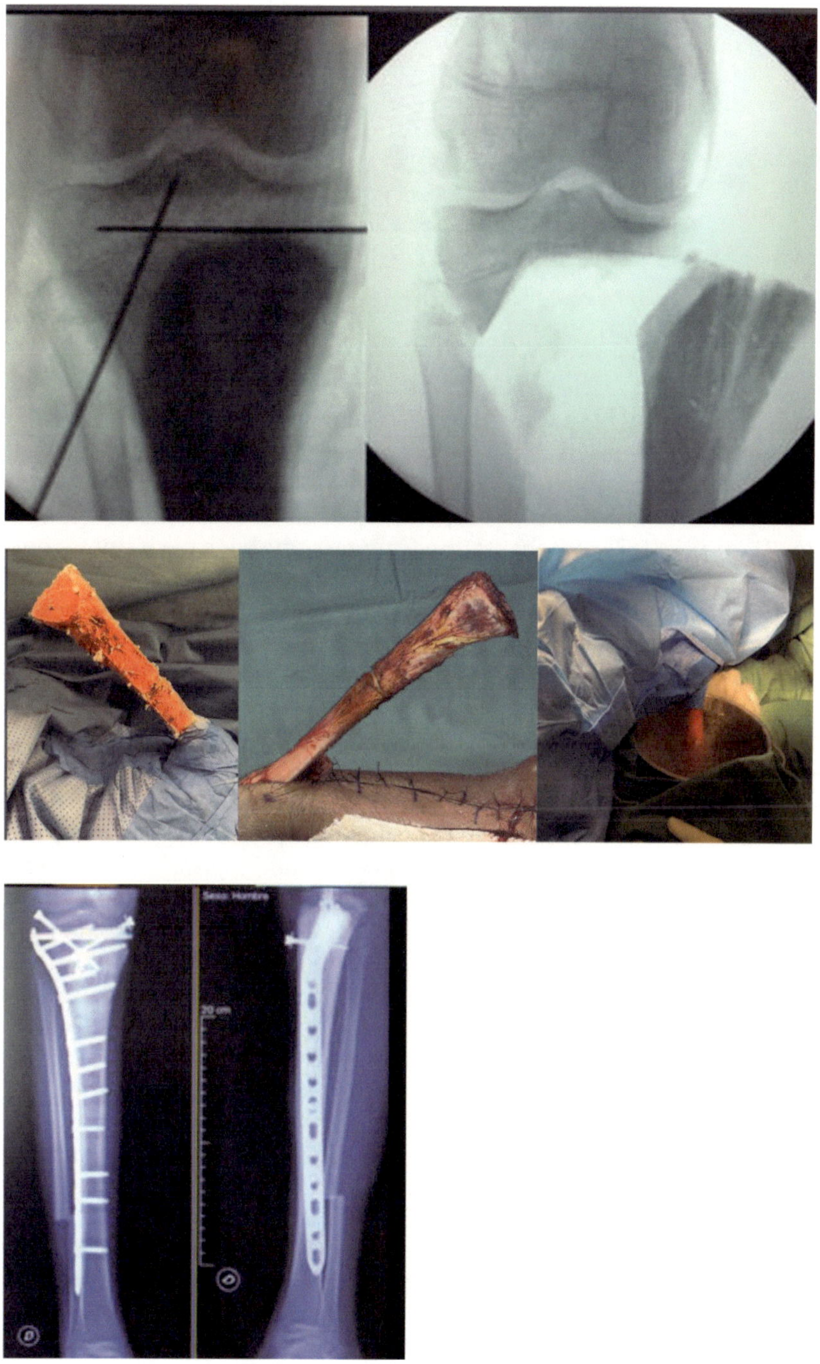

Figure 7.
Case of a 15-year-old male with an osteoblastic osteosarcoma abutting the proximal tibial physis, treated with limb salvage surgery with liquid nitrogen pretreated bone tumor autograft. Careful surgical planning allowed the proximal physis to be preserved.

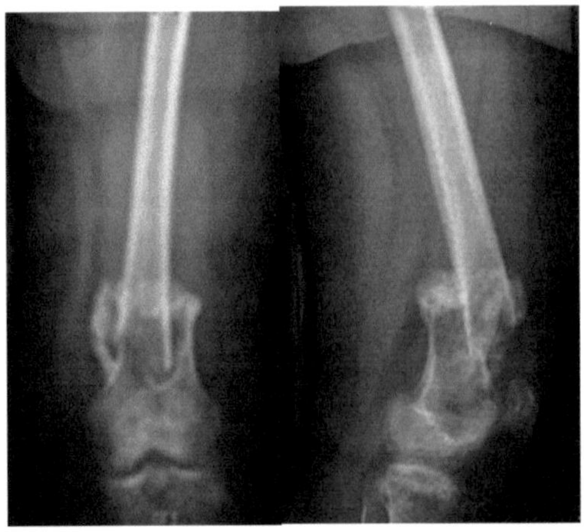

Figure 8.
Radiographic image depicting a pathological fracture through a distal femur osteosarcoma with displacement and shortening of the distal fragment.

Frozen autografts recycled in liquid nitrogen are a biologic solution with the advantages of low cost, easy access, complete removal of viable tumor, bone morphogenic protein preservation, osteoconduction and osteoinduction properties maintained, perfect matching at the osteotomy site, does not require a bone bank, allows reattachment of tendons and ligaments, no disease transmission and no graft rejection (**Figure 7**) [47]. Among its disadvantages, the bone piece cannot be sent for full pathology analysis and thus provide the information about the percentage of necrosis obtained after systemic treatment in the indicated cases. Nonetheless, the surrounding soft tissues which are resected prior to submerging the piece in LN are sent to pathology. This technique accomplishes full necrosis of the tumoral cells and prior studies have shown that the soft tissue resection prior to the sterilization in LN is representative of the tumor response to chemotherapy [48]. Additionally, this procedure has shown no difference in terms of bone resistance to compression when compared to unfrozen bone. This allows for the initial resistance of the reconstruction, being comparable or even superior to allografts [48].

One particular scenario, the treating orthopedic oncologist should be aware of is the case of an osteosarcoma with a pathological fracture at presentation. Fractures through an osteogenic sarcoma can occur in up to 10% of the cases (**Figure 8**) [14]. In the past, this circumstance used to be a contraindication for a limb salvage procedure and patients were indisputably recommended for an amputation. Nowadays, even though those patients tend to present a worse prognosis, a limb salvage procedure is considered an option with similar recurrence rates when compared to amputations [49]. Prior studies presented the hypothesis that these patients may have a worse outcome due to a hematoma formation at the fracture site, with tumor cell dissemination [50]. Although the ideal treatment is controversial, some authors recommend stabilization of the fracture, which could be achieved by casting, external fixation or limited internal fixation followed by neoadjuvant chemotherapy, subsequent definite surgical treatment and adjuvant systemic treatment [51, 52].

Radiotherapy has a role for unresectable tumors or in cases of positive margins to help with local control. The Cooperative Osteosarcoma Study Group (COSS) has presented promising results for the case of unresectable osteosarcomas of the spine and pelvis where the treatment with radiation with a curative intent improved the 5-year survival from 0 to 29% [53, 54]. Additional studies have shown radiation is well tolerated by the patients and can achieve up to 76% local control rates [55]. These findings seem to indicate osteosarcomas do have at least a moderate response to radiotherapy, when in the past it used to be considered a radiotherapy resistant tumor. Supplementary indications for radiotherapy include symptom palliation and this treatment modality has shown to improve patients' symptoms such as pain in case of unresectable tumors [56].

Current investigation trials are in place to uncover targetable mutations that could also have prognostic implications as well studies to assess a potential role for immunotherapy in osteosarcoma patients [57]. Specifically, Cabozantinib, a tyrosine kinase inhibitor used for thyroid and renal cell cancers, has shown anti-tumor activity as well as a good tolerance and is currently under investigation through multicentre trials [58].

5. Conclusion

Osteosarcoma, the most common primary bone malignancy in children and adolescents, has come a long way since its initial approach where all patients underwent an amputation prior to the 1970's. Current systemic treatment options along the myriad of reconstruction alternatives, have allowed these patients to benefit from better survival rates and improved function and quality of life. Nonetheless, the overall survival rates have remained stable for the past 50 years, a disappointing number when compared to other malignancies' statistics, suggesting more resources and research are needed to continue enhancing the outcomes of patients suffering from this cancer.

Conflict of interest

The authors state no conflict of interest related to the writing of this chapter.

Author details

Gottardo Bianchi[1], Leticia Gaiero[1], Nicolas Casales[1], Claudio Silveri[1] and Ana C. Belzarena[2*]

1 Oncology Orthopedic Department, University of the Republic, Montevideo, Uruguay

2 Oncology Orthopedic Service, Miami Cancer Institute, Baptist Health South Florida, Miami, Florida, United States

*Address all correspondence to: ceciliabel@baptisthealth.net

References

[1] Anderson ME. Update on survival in osteosarcoma, Orthop. Clin. North Am. 47 (1) (2016) 283e292.S.

[2] Mutsaers AJ, Walkley CR. Cells of origin in osteosarcoma: mesenchymal stem cells or osteoblast committed cells?. Bone. 2014;62:56-63. doi:10.1016/j.bone.2014.02.003.

[3] Key Statistics for Osteosarcoma. (n.d.). Retrieved February 01, 2021, from https://www.cancer.org/cancer/osteosarcoma/about/key-statistics.html

[4] Cotterill SJ, Wright CM, Pearce MS, Craft AW. Stature of young people with malignant bone tumors. Pediatr Blood Cancer. 2004;42:59-63. doi: 10.1002/pbc.10437.

[5] Pan Y, Chen D, Hu T, Lv G, Dai Z. Characteristics and Prognostic Factors of Patients With Osteosarcoma Older Than 60 Years From the SEER Database. Cancer Control. 2019;26(1):1073274819888893. doi:10.1177/1073274819888893.

[6] Toki S, Kobayashi E, Yoshida A, et al. A clinical comparison between dedifferentiated low-grade osteosarcoma and conventional osteosarcoma. Bone Joint J. 2019;101-B(6):745-752. doi:10.1302/0301-620X.101B6.BJJ-2018-1207.R1.

[7] Shimatani A, Aono M, Hoshi M, et al. Secondary osteosarcoma in patients previously treated for childhood cancer: Three case reports. Mol Clin Oncol. 2019;10(1):153-158. doi:10.3892/mco.2018.1752.

[8] Martin JW, Squire JA, Zielenska M. The genetics of osteosarcoma. Sarcoma. 2012;2012:627254.

[9] Morrow JJ, Khanna C. Osteosarcoma Genetics and Epigenetics: Emerging Biology and Candidate Therapies. Crit Rev Oncog. 2015;20(3-4):173-197. doi:10.1615/critrevoncog.2015013713.

[10] Bielack SS, Kempf-Bielack B, Delling G, et al. Prognostic factors in high-grade osteosarcoma of the extremities or trunk: An analysis of 1,702 patients treated on neoadjuvant cooperative osteosarcoma study group protocols. J Clin Oncol. 2002;20:776-790.

[11] Kawai A, Huvos AG, Meyers PA, Healey JH, Osteosarcoma of the pelvis. Oncologic results of 40 patients, Clin. Orthop. Relat. Res. 348 (1998)196e207.

[12] Han I, Lee YM, Cho HS, Oh JH, Lee SH, Kim HS. Outcome after surgical treatment of pelvic sarcomas, Clin. Orthop. Surg. 2 (3) (2010) 160e166.

[13] Reed DR, Hayashi M, Wagner L, et al. Treatment pathway of bone sarcoma in children, adolescents, and young adults. Cancer. 2017;123(12):2206-2218. doi:10.1002/cncr.30589.

[14] Lozano Calderón SA, Garbutt C, Kim J, et al. Clinical and Molecular Analysis of Pathologic Fracture-associated Osteosarcoma: MicroRNA profile Is Different and Correlates with Prognosis. Clin Orthop Relat Res. 2019;477(9):2114-2126. doi:10.1097/CORR.0000000000000867.

[15] Zhang C, Guo X, Xu Y, et al. Lung metastases at the initial diagnosis of high-grade osteosarcoma: prevalence, risk factors and prognostic factors. A large population-based cohort study. Sao Paulo Med J. 2019;137(5):423-429. doi:10.1590/1516-3180.2018.0381120619.

[16] Kumar R, Kumar M, Malhotra K, Patel S. Primary osteosarcoma in the elderly revisited: current concepts in

diagnosis and treatment. Curr Oncol Rep. 2018;20(2):13.

[17] Longhi A, Errani C, Gonzales-Arabio D, Ferrari C, Mercuri M. Osteosarcoma in patients older than 65 years. J Clin Oncol. 2008;26(33):5368-5373.

[18] Nishida Y, Isu K, Ueda T, et al. Osteosarcoma in the elderly over 60 years: a multicenter study by the Japanese Musculoskeletal Oncology Group. J Surg Oncol. 2009;100(1):48-54.

[19] Kundu ZS. Classification, imaging, biopsy and staging of osteosarcoma. Indian J Orthop. 2014;48(3):238-246. doi:10.4103/0019-5413.132491.

[20] Morrison WB, Dalinka MK, Daffner RH, et al. Bone tumors. In: ACR appropriateness criteria. Reston, VA: American College of Radiology, 2005:1-5.

[21] Resnick D. Tumors and tumor-like lesions of bone: radiographic principles. In: Resnick D, ed. Diagnosis of bone and joint disorders. Philadelphia, PA: Saunders, 2002:3745-3762.

[22] Rubin DA. Magnetic resonance imaging: Practical considerations. In: Resnick D, Kransdorf MJ, editors. Bone and joint imaging. 3rd ed. Philadelphia Pennsylvania: Elsevier Saunders; 2005. pp. 118-32.

[23] Mankin HJ, Mankin CJ, Simon MA. The hazards of biopsy, revisited: Members of Musculoskeletal Society. J Bone Joint Surg. 1996;64:656-63.

[24] Meyers PA, Heller G, Healey JH, et al. Osteogenic sarcoma with clinically detectable metastasis at initial presentation. J Clin Oncol. 1993;11(3):449-53. PMID: 8445419; doi: 10.1200/JCO.1993.11.3.449.

[25] Kager L, Zoubek A, Pötschger U, et al. Primary metastatic osteosarcoma: presentation and outcome of patients treated on neoadjuvant Cooperative Osteosarcoma Study Group protocols. J Clin Oncol. 2003;21(10):2011-8. PMID: 12743156; doi: 10.1200/JCO.2003.08.132.

[26] Bacci G, Longhi A, Bertoni F, et al. Bone metastases in osteosarcoma patients treated with neoadjuvant or adjuvant chemotherapy: the Rizzoli experience in 52 patients. Acta Orthop. 2006;77(6):938-943. doi:10.1080/17453670610013268.

[27] Isakoff MS, Bielack SS, Meltzer P, Gorlick R. Osteosarcoma: Current Treatment and a Collaborative Pathway to Success. Journal of clinical oncology : official journal of the American Society of Clinical Oncology. 2015; 33:3029-35.

[28] Hoshi M, Takami M, Ieguchi M, et al. Fertility following treatment of high-grade malignant bone and soft tissue tumors in young adults. Mol Clin Oncol. 2015;3(2):367-374. doi:10.3892/mco.2014.474.

[29] Gorlick R, Khanna C. Osteosarcoma. J Bone Miner Res. 2010; 25:683-91.

[30] Marina N, Gebhardt M, Teot L, Gorlick R. Biology and therapeutic advances for pediatric osteosarcoma. Oncologist. 2004;9(4):422-441.

[31] Chen R, Wang G, Zheng Y, Hua Y, Cai Z. Drug resistance-related microRNAs in osteosarcoma: Translating basic evidence into therapeutic strategies. J Cell Mol Med. 2019;23(4):2280-2292. doi:10.1111/jcmm.14064.

[32] Goorin AM, Schwartzentruber DJ, Devidas M, et al. Presurgical chemotherapy compared with immediate surgery and adjuvant chemotherapy for nonmetastatic osteosarcoma: Pediatric Oncology Group Study POG-8651. J Clin Oncol. 2003;21:1574-1580.

[33] Picci P, Sangiorgi L, Rougraff BT, Neff JR, Casadei R, Campanacci M. Relationship of chemotherapy-induced necrosis and surgical margins to local recurrence in osteosarcoma. J Clin Oncol. 1994;12(12):2699-2705. doi:10.1200/JCO.1994.12.12.2699.

[34] Marulanda GA, Henderson ER, Johnson DA, Letson GD, Cheong D. Orthopedic surgery options for the treatment of primary osteosarcoma. Cancer Control. 2008;15(1):13-20. doi:10.1177/107327480801500103.

[35] Aksnes LH, Bauer HC, Jebsen NL, et al. Limb-sparing surgery preserves more function than amputation: a Scandinavian sarcoma group study of 118 patients. J Bone Joint Surg Br. 2008;90(6):786-794. doi:10.1302/0301-620X.90B6.19805.

[36] Jeys LM, Thorne CJ, Parry M, Gaston CL, Sumathi VP, Grimer JR. A Novel System for the Surgical Staging of Primary High-grade Osteosarcoma: The Birmingham Classification. Clin Orthop Relat Res. 2017;475(3):842-850. doi:10.1007/s11999-016-4851-y.

[37] Cates JM. Reporting Surgical Resection Margin Status for Osteosarcoma: Comparison of the AJCC, MSTS, and Margin Distance Methods. Am J Surg Pathol. 2017;41(5):633-642. doi:10.1097/PAS.0000000000000815.

[38] Takeuchi A, Lewis VO, Satcher RL, Moon BS, Lin PP. What are the factors that affect survival and relapse after local recurrence of osteosarcoma?. Clin Orthop Relat Res. 2014;472(10):3188-3195. doi:10.1007/s11999-014-3759-7.

[39] Frisoni T, Cevolani L, Giorgini A, et al. Factors affecting outcome of massive intercalary bone allografts in the treatment of tumours of the femur. J Bone Joint Surg. 2012; 94:836-41.

[40] Mankin HJ, Gebhardt MC, Jennings LC, et al. Long-term results of allograft replacement in the management of bone tumors. Clin Orthop Relat Res. 1996; 324: 86-97.

[41] Donati D, Colangeli M, Colangeli S, et al. Allograft-prosthetic composite in the proximal tibia after bone tumor resection. Clin Orthop Relat Res. 2008; 466:459-65.

[42] Yajima, H, Tamai S, Mizumoto S et al. Vascularized fibular grafts for reconstruction of the femur. J Bone Joint Surg. 1993; 75: 123-28.

[43] Watanabe K, Tsuchiya H, Yamamoto N, et al. Over 10-year follow-up of functional outcome in patients with bone tumors reconstructed using distraction osteogenesis. J Orthop Sci. 2013; 18:101-09.

[44] Tsuchiya H, Tomita K. Reconstruction using an autograft containing tumour treated by liquid nitrogen. J Bone Joint Surg Br. 2005; 87:218-25.

[45] Torbert JT, Fox EJ, Hosalkar HS, et al. Endoprosthetic reconstructions: results of long-term follow up of 139 patients. Clin Orthop Relat Res. 2005; 438:51-9.

[46] Tomford WW. Transmission of disease through transplantation of musculoskeletal allografts. J Bone Joint Surg Am. 1995; 77(11): 1742-54.

[47] Takata M, Sugimoto N, Yamamoto N, et al. Activity of bone morphogenetic protein-7 after treatment at various temperatures: freezing vs. pasteurization vs. allograft. Cryobiology. 2011; 63:235-39.

[48] Yamamoto N, Tsuchiya H, Tomita K. Effects of liquid nitrogen treatment on the proliferation of osteosarcoma and the biomechanical properties of normal bone. J Orthop Sci. 2003; 8:374-80.

[49] Bacci G, Ferrari S, Longhi A, Donati D, Manfrini M, Giacomini S, Briccoli A, Forni C, Galletti S. Nonmetastatic osteosarcoma of the extremity with pathologic fracture at presentation: local and systemic control by amputation or limb salvage after preoperative chemotherapy. Acta Orthop Scand. 2003;74:449-454.

[50] Abudu A, Sferopoulos NK, Tillman RM, Carter SR, Grimer RJ. The surgical treatment and outcome of pathological fractures in localised osteosarcoma. J Bone Joint Surg Br. 1996;78(5):694-698.

[51] Scully SP, Ghert MA, Zurakowski D, Thompson RC, Gebhardt MC. Pathologic fracture in osteosarcoma : prognostic importance and treatment implications [published correction appears in J Bone Joint Surg Am 2002 Apr;84-A(4):622]. J Bone Joint Surg Am. 2002;84(1):49-57.

[52] Scully SP, Temple HT, O'Keefe RJ, Mankin HJ, Gebhardt M. The surgical treatment of patients with osteosarcoma who sustain a pathologic fracture. Clin Orthop Relat Res. 1996;(324):227-232. doi:10.1097/00003086-199603000-00028.

[53] Ozaki T, Flege S, Kevric M, et al. Osteosarcoma of the pelvis: experience of the Cooperative Osteosarcoma Study Group. J Clin Oncol 2003;21(2):334-341.

[54] Ozaki T, Flege S, Liljenqvist U, et al. Osteosarcoma of the spine: experience of the Cooperative Osteosarcoma Study Group. Cancer 2002;94(4):1069-1077.

[55] Tinkle CL, Lu J, Han Y, et al. Curative-intent radiotherapy for pediatric osteosarcoma: The St. Jude experience. Pediatr Blood Cancer. 2019;66(8):e27763. doi:10.1002/pbc.27763.

[56] Mahajan A, Woo SY, Kornguth DG, et al. Multimodality treatment of osteosarcoma: radiation in a high-risk cohort. Pediatr. Blood Cancer 2008;50(5):976-982.

[57] Bishop MW, Janeway KA, Gorlick R. Future directions in the treatment of osteosarcoma. Curr Opin Pediatr. 2016;28(1):26-33. doi:10.1097/MOP.0000000000000298.

[58] Italiano A, Mir O, Mathoulin-Pelissier S, et al. Cabozantinib in patients with advanced Ewing sarcoma or osteosarcoma (CABONE): a multicentre, single-arm, phase 2 trial. Lancet Oncol. 2020;21(3):446-455. doi:10.1016/S1470-2045(19)30825-3.

Chapter 5

Current Therapeutic Approaches for Osteosarcoma

Recep Öztürk

Abstract

Osteosarcoma is classically defined as a high-grade spindle-shaped neoplasm with malignant cells that produce osteoid. It is the most common primary malignant bone tumor in children and young adults. It is <1% of all cancers diagnosed, approximately 3.4% of all childhood cancers. The age-adjusted incidence of osteosarcoma is bimodal, with an initial peak in adolescence and then a second peak in patients over 60 years of age. Osteosarcoma is divided into two main groups. In most of the osteosarcomas, the etiological agent cannot be determined and it is called primary osteosarcoma. Osteosarcoma, which develops due to etiologies such as Paget's disease, radiotherapy or osteonecrosis, is called seconder osteosarcoma. Osteosarcomas are most commonly located in the appendicular skeleton. The most common settlement here is the knee circumference. The distal femur and proximal tibia are the most common locations in the knee. A multidisciplinary approach is indicated in the management of osteosarcoma. The treatment is multimodal, including systemic chemotherapy and local therapy. In this section, we will outline the current standard of care for the systemic and surgical approach to osteosarcoma treatment, as well as an overview of current studies.

Keywords: osteosarcoma, recent advances, management, current approach, treatment

1. Introduction

Osteosarcoma is the most common primary malignant bone tumor. It consists of malignant mesenchymal cells that tend to form osteoid matter. It is defined as the most common bone malignant tumor after multiple myeloma and metastases [1, 2].

Three-quarters of all cases are between the ages of 10–25. The age-adjusted incidence of osteosarcoma is bimodal, with an initial peak in adolescence and then a second peak in patients over 60 years of age [3].

Osteosarcoma is most often located around the knee. Distal femur and proximal tibia are the most common knee localizations. The most common location after knee circumference is the proximal humerus. The most common location of the tumor in the bone is the metaphysis like many other tumors. It can rarely settle in the diaphysis [4].

2. Etiology and risk factors

In osteosarcoma cases in pediatric patients, almost all cases do not have any identifiable associated risk factors.

IntechOpen

It has been determined that in almost half of the osteosarcoma cases seen in adult patients, various risk factors such as Paget's disease and radiation are involved in the etiology. In addition, some syndromes such as Li Fraumeni Syndrome, hereditary retinoblastoma syndrome, have been reported as risk factors for osteosarcoma [5].

Studies have been conducted on the genetic profile of osteosarcoma in recent years. Studies have reported that Germline TP53 mutations may be high in osteosarcomas, especially at younger ages. In osteosarcomas seen at a young age, if the location of the tumor is unusual, further examination is recommended in terms of Li-Fraumeni syndrome [6].

3. Classification

Osteosarcoma is divided into two main groups as primary and secondary osteosarcoma. Primary osteosarcoma is divided into subtypes such as classical osteosarcoma, telangiectatic osteosarcoma, small cell osteosarcoma, multicentric osteosarcoma, high grade central osteosarcoma, low gradesurface osteosarcoma, and superficial (parosteal-periosteal) osteosarcoma [7].

Various etiological factors play a role in secondary osteosarcoma. Osteosarcoma secondary to Paget's disease, osteosarcoma secondary to radiotherapy, osteosarcoma secondary to osteonecrosis, osteosarcoma secondary to fibrous dysplasia are some of the secondary osteosarcoma types [5].

4. Clinical findings and diagnosis

The most common clinical finding is pain and is seen in approximately 90% of patients. The second most common finding is swelling in the bone localization and is detected in approximately 50% of cases. Generally, patients present with complaints of pain and swelling in that area for weeks-months. Another finding is limitation of movement and is seen in approximately 45% of cases. In addition, patients rarely present with pathological fractures (about 8%) [8].

Alkaline phosphatase was found to be high in about half of osteosarcoma patients. High levels of lactate dehydrogenase at the time of diagnosis were found to be associated with relapse. In addition, Lactate dehydrogenase levels are also high in metastatic patients [8, 9].

In radiological evaluation, firstly, anteroposterior and lateral radiographs of the relevant region should be taken (**Figure 1**). When direct X-ray findings, bone involving the lesion, location of the tumor in the bone, age and gender of the patient are evaluated together, a correct diagnosis can be made in most of the cases (more than three quarters of the cases) [10].

Cortex destruction, geographic or moth-eaten-like medullary lesion, sunlight-like periosteal reaction, Codman triangle, and soft tissue shadow in the bone neighborhood can be seen on plain X-ray [11].

Whenever there is any doubt about the nature of a bone lesion in a young patient, CT and/or MRI should be performed. Thus, new bone formation, cortical destruction, or soft tissue component that may indicate malignancy can be detected (**Figure 2**). In addition to imaging the primary tumor, MRI should be taken to view the entire bone to detect possible skip metastases [12].

Performing the MRI test before any biopsy attempt is vital, as reactive changes due to biopsy reduce staging accuracy [13].

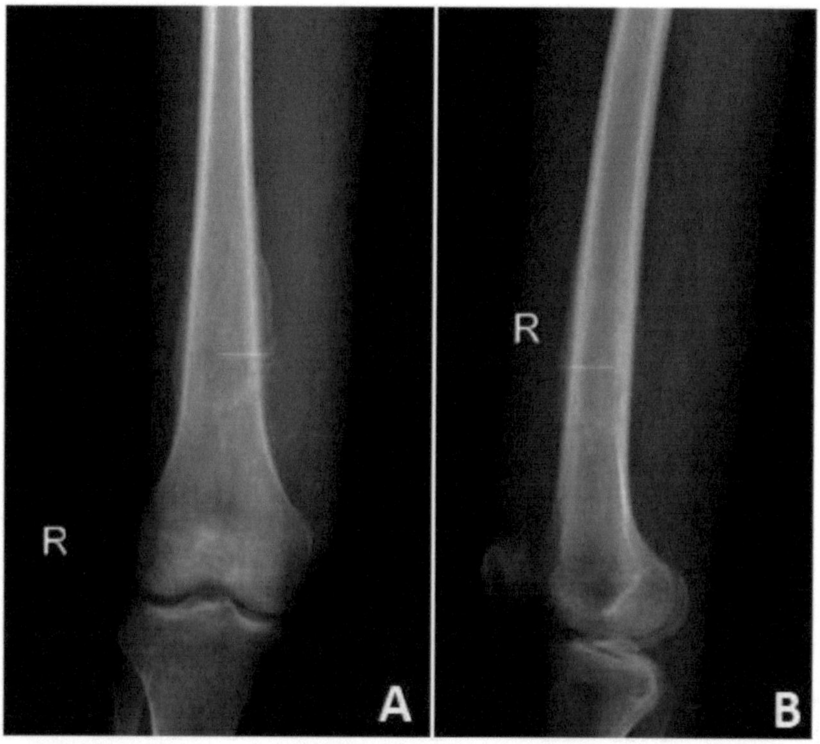

Figure 1.
Right femur distal located osteosarcoma, a) anteroposterior and b) lateral radiography.

Radiological examinations are examined for the presence of findings specific to malignant bone tumors. These findings are sclerotic lesions that are located mostly in the metaphysis, progressing towards the epiphysis or diaphysis or laterally, radial calcified areas, disruption of the cortex integrity, fragmentation or elevation of the periosteum, Codman triangle and extension of the lesion to the soft tissue [11, 14].

The definitive diagnosis is made after the histopathological examination of the biopsy specimen. Biopsy should be done by the team that will make the definitive treatment of the patient. The formation of osteoid material and the presence of atypical osteoblasts are diagnostic. CT-assisted needle biopsies and, if necessary, incisional biopsy should be performed in the trace of the original surgical incision [2].

5. Staging

Osteosarcoma is considered a systemic disease. Tumor cells are present in the circulating blood and tumor micro-metastases are possible in the lungs. Approximately 10–20% of osteosarcoma patients are metastatic at the time of diagnosis [15].

It is a three-grade system generally used in determining tumor grade. Grade 1 represents low grade. There is a well-differentiated tumor. Grade 2 represents middle grade, there is a moderately differentiated tumor. Grade 3 represents high grade, there is an undifferentiated tumor. If the tumor grade is low, the tumor is resistant to chemotherapy and radiotherapy [2, 7].

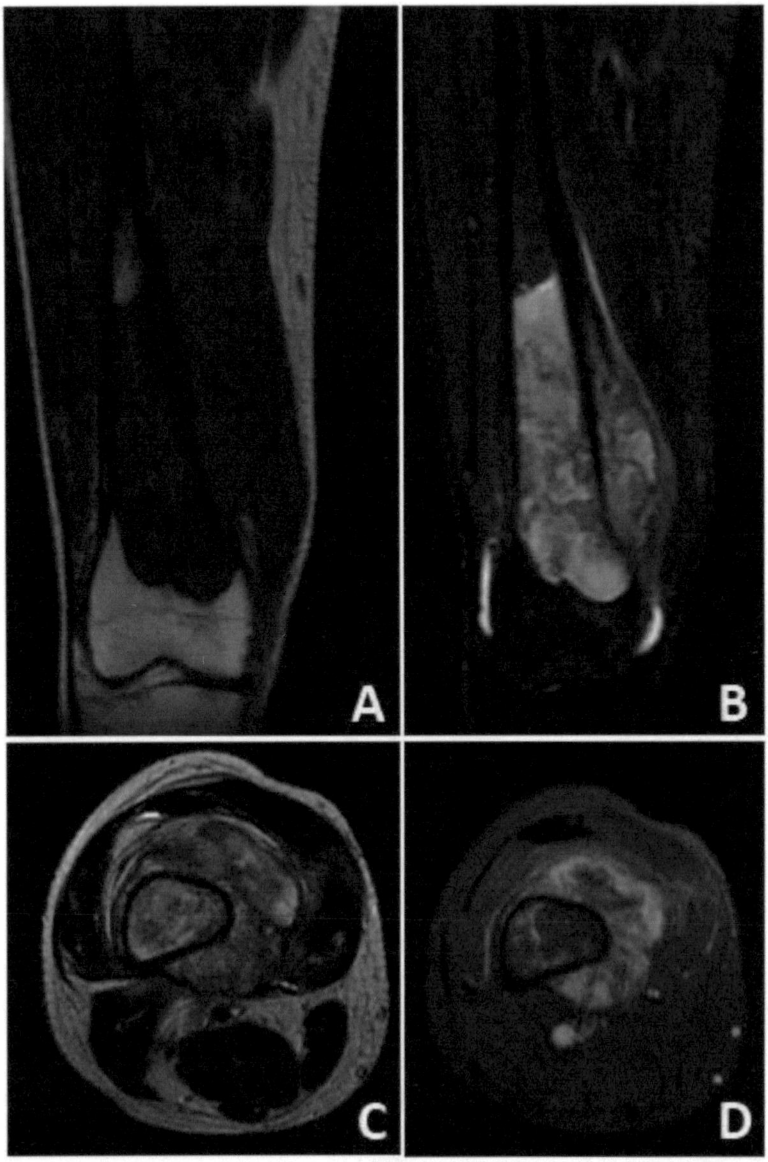

Figure 2.
MRI images involving the right femur distal and joint; a) coronal T1 sequence, b) coronal T2 - STIR image, c) axial T2 sequence and d) T1 + contrast image. In the images, the distal third of the right femur has an extension to the superior part of the inner femoral condyle and the midline distal of the femur, and has a satellite nodular structure of approximately 5.5 mm in the epiphyseal line, especially in the T1A series, the heterogeneous hyperintense signal in the T2A series, infiltrating bone marrow fat 12.5 there is a mass lesion of x4cm. Especially when T2 sequence was examined, it was determined that the mass showed extra cortical and extra osseous spread in the inner part, periosteal reaction and accompanying a soft tissue mass in the intramuscular localization with an intramuscular localization of approximately 84x48mm with a heterogeneous necrotic contrast in the soft tissue. Low-intensity, especially peripherally wavy rim-style contrast enhancement was noted in post-contrast series.

Osteosarcoma most often metastasizes to the lungs. This is followed by bone metastases. Contrast-enhanced thin-section CT of the lung is the gold standard in detecting the presence of metastasis in the lung. Skip metastases in the same bone and distant bone metastases can be detected by Whole-Body Bone Scintigraphy. PET-CT is valuable in showing all body metastases and evaluating the chemotherapy response after treatment. Also useful for detecting nucleus [7, 8, 11].

6. Treatment management

In the past, patients with osteosarcoma were tried to be treated with amputation, but patients were lost due to micro-metastatic disease and lung metastases. With the discovery that chemotherapy can eliminate micro-metastases (1970's), limb-sparing surgeries came to the fore [16]. The application of neoadjuvant chemotherapy and limb-sparing surgeries became standard in the 1980s. This paved the way for the development of limb salvage procedures that can achieve limb with better functional and cosmetic results. With the advances in treatment, studies on long-term functional and cosmetic extremity acquisition methods have increased.

With the development of induction and adjuvant chemotherapy protocols and advances in surgical techniques and radiological staging studies, approximately 90–95% of patients are now treated with limb-sparing methods instead of amputation. In limb-sparing surgery, reconstruction is applied in necessary patients in addition to tumor resection. And after all these advances, the chance of long-term survival and cure rate of these patients increased to 60–80% in localized (non-metastatic) diseases [17].

In classical osteosarcoma, the general treatment plan is preoperative (neoadjuvant) chemotherapy, extremity conserving surgery if possible, and postoperative chemotherapy regimen based on the extent of tumor necrosis. In surgical treatment, the tumor is resected with wide margins. Amputation is performed for patients who cannot undergo limb-sparing surgery [18]. Osteosarcoma is a radioresistant tumor and radiotherapy does not have therapeutic properties.

The high-dose methotrexate with leucovorin rescue (HDMTX), doxorubicin and cisplatin (MAP) trio is the basis of standard systemic chemotherapy and is administered for approximately 30 weeks [16]. In a newly diagnosed osteosarcoma patient, 2 cycles of neoadjuvant chemotherapy (2 MAP cycles for approximately 10 weeks) are applied first.

After the HDMTX infusion administered for 2 weeks, a 1-week break is taken, then doxorubicin and cisplatin are administered for 2 days. And a 2-week break is given for bone marrow recovery. And the cycle repeats. Then, surgical treatment is applied [19].

Histological response value evaluated during surgical treatment is a strong prognostic factor. High tumor necrosis rate has better clinical outcomes after neoadjuvant chemotherapy [20].

The results of surgery alone are very poor in osteosarcoma treatment. And with chemotherapy alone, only about 10% of the patients responded [21].

Local control can be achieved through limb salvage surgery or ablative surgery (**Figure 3**). There is no significant difference between amputation and wide resection in local surgery in terms of recurrence and survival rates. Metastasectomy should be considered in lung metastases [14].

In recent years, many studies have been conducted on reconstruction after tumor resection with wide margins in local treatment and reconstruction options have been diversified. Custom-made or modular tumor resection prostheses are one of them. In addition, osteoarticular allografts and composite allografts are other options. With the advances in microsurgery, vascular fibula and myo-cutaneous flaps have also become an alternative for reconstruction. Another option is the method of recovered bone (reconstruction of the bone with the tumor tissue covered by removing the tumor, autoclaving or irradiating it or treating the bone with liquid nitrogen) [11, 22].

After the HDMTX infusion administered for 2 weeks, a 1-week break is given, then doxorubicin and cisplatin are administered for 2 days. And a 2-week break is

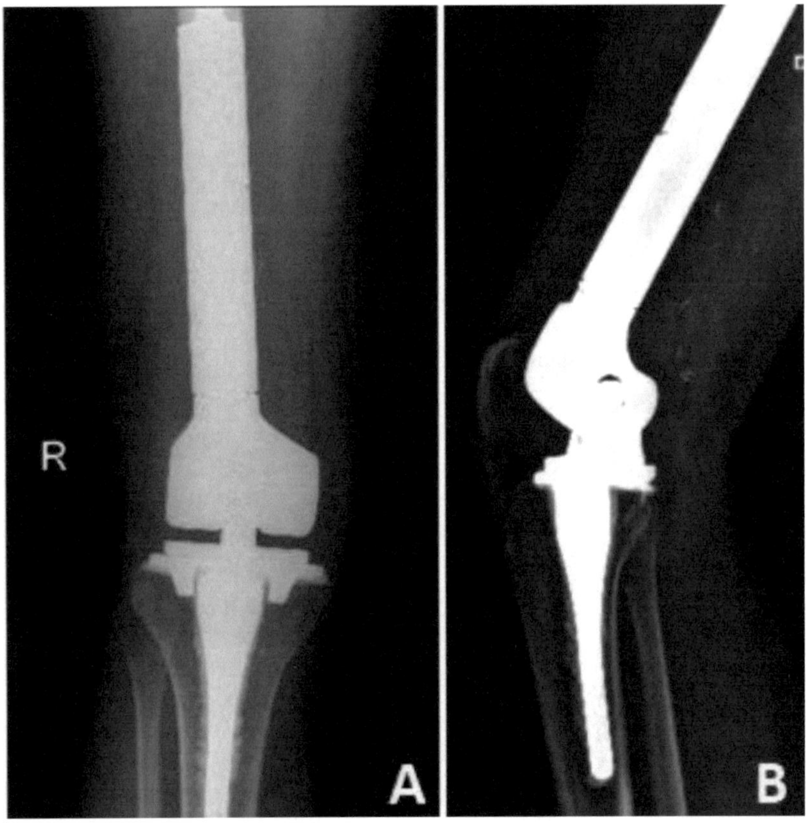

Figure 3.
Right femur distal located osteosarcoma, post-operatively a) anteroposterior and b) lateral radiography. There was skip metastasis in the epiphysis localization of the distal femur. Tumor resection with white margins and reconstruction operation with distal femur tumor resection prosthesis were performed as local treatment.

given for bone marrow recovery. And the cycle repeats. Then, surgical treatment is applied [16].

Overall survival for lower limb reconstructions ranges from about 70–85% at 5 years [23].

Adjuvant MAP therapy should be initiated within 3 weeks after surgical treatment. Because especially in patients with low tumor necrosis rate, a delay of more than 3 weeks is associated with high recurrence rates. Current standard adjuvant chemotherapy includes a total of 29 weeks of MAP cycles.

7. Prognosis

Several prognostic factors have been identified in the management and follow-up of osteosarcoma. Stage (local-systemic spread) is a poor prognostic factor. As the tumor stage increases, the prognosis worsens. Another prognostic factor is tumor grade. Low grade types are parosteal osteosarcoma, periosteal osteosarcoma and low-grade intramedullary osteosarcoma. Tumor size is poor prognostic. As the tumor size increases, the prognosis worsens. Tumor localization affects the prognosis. Tumors located distal to the elbow in the upper extremity and tumors located distal to the knee in the lower extremity have a relatively better prognosis. It has been reported that the presence of pathological fractures does not affect the prognosis. Gender has also been reported as a prognostic factor. The prognosis is relatively better in female patients. Prognosis is worse in secondary osteosarcoma. Five-year survival is less than 10% in osteosarcoma patients developing on the basis of Paget's disease, and 5-year survival is less than 20% in patients with osteosarcoma developing on a radiation background [11, 14, 24]. The presence of metastatic disease is another poor prognostic factor.

Patients should be followed for at least five years in terms of systemic metastases postoperatively.

In patients with macro-metastasis at the time of diagnosis, despite systemic chemotherapy and surgery, 5-year disease-free survival is approximately 20% [25]. In addition, 10-year survival is less than 20% in relapse cases [26].

8. Recent advances

Studies on intensified chemotherapy are continuing in patients who underwent surgery after neoadjuvant chemotherapy and in patients with poor histological response detected during surgery. Poor histological responders are defined as patients who maintain more than 10% viable tumors following surgery. Current studies report that chemotherapy intensification has less successful results than thought [20, 27].

Several clinical studies have been investigating the intensification of adjuvant chemotherapy by adding high-dose ifosfamide with or without etoposide to MAP for poor histological responders following definitive surgery. However, it has not been shown to be superior to standard chemotherapy. In addition, studies with cytokine interferon alfa-2b showed that this agent did not provide superiority to standard therapy [20, 27].

Studies with high-dose ifosfamide to avoid the long-term nephrotoxic effects of methotrexate have shown equivalent effect rates [28]. Similarly, studies have been conducted with dexrazoxane to avoid long-term nephrotoxic effects of doxorubicin. [29].

9. Conclusions

The current standard of care for a patient with newly diagnosed osteosarcoma includes 2 cycles of MAP neoadjuvant chemotherapy followed by local tumor surgery and 29 weeks of adjuvant MAP chemotherapy. With this standard approach, disease-free survival is approximately 70% in patients with localized disease at the time of diagnosis.

Treatment outcomes for patients with osteosarcoma, for localized, metastatic, or relapse patients, have not improved significantly and have not gotten better in the last 10 years, despite many improvements and extensive studies.

The poor results of patients with low necrosis during surgery after neoadjuvant chemotherapy still appear as a treatment challenge. It has been shown that intensified chemotherapy methods, which have been emphasized in recent years, are not superior to conventional treatment. It is clear that more work is needed.

Conflict of interest

The authors declare no conflict of interest.

Author details

Recep Öztürk
Dr. Abdurrahman Yurtaslan Ankara Oncology Training and Research Hospital, Ankara, Turkey

*Address all correspondence to: ozturk_recep@windowslive.com

References

[1] Whelan JS. Osteosarcoma. Eur J Cancer. 1997;33(10):1611-1618; discussion 1618-9. DOI: 10.1016/s0959-8049(97)00251-7.

[2] Mirra JM. Malignant Bone Tumours. In: Mirra JM, Picci P, Gold RH. Bone Tumours: Clinical, Radiologic, and Pathologic Correlations, Philadelphia: Lea and Febiger; 1989. p.248-389.

[3] Mirabello L, Troisi RJ, Savage SA. International osteosarcoma incidence patterns in children and adolescents, middle ages and elderly persons. Int J Cancer. 2009 Jul;125(1):229-234. DOI: 10.1002/ijc.24320.

[4] Öztürk R, İnce B, Karakoç Y, Arıkan ŞM, Yapar AE, Erdoğdu Yİ, et al. Evaluation of Demographic and Clinicopathological Characteristics of Osteosarcoma Patients. Acta Oncol Tur. 2019;52(2):266-270. DOI: 10.5505/aot.2019.60234.

[5] Fuchs B, Pritchard DJ. Etiology of osteosarcoma. Clin OrthopRelat Res. 2002;(397):40-52. DOI: 10.1097/00003086-200204000-00007.

[6] Mirabello L, Yeager M, Mai PL, Gastier-Foster JM, Gorlick R, Khanna C, et al.. Germline TP53 variants and susceptibility to osteosarcoma. J Natl Cancer Inst. 2015;107(7):djv101. DOI: 10.1093/jnci/djv101.

[7] Greanspan A, Jundt G, Remagen W. Differential Diagnosis in Orthopaedic Oncology. Bone Forming (Osteogenic) Lesions. 2nd ed. Philadelphia: Lippincott Williams & Wilkins; 2007. p.88-9.

[8] Greenspan A. Orthopedic Imaging. 4th ed. California, Lippincott Williams& Wilkins. 2005; 689-696.

[9] Link MP, Goorin AM, Horowitz M, Meyer WH, Belasco J, Baker A, et al. Adjuvant chemotherapy of high-grade osteosarcoma of the extremity. Updated results of the Multi-Institutional Osteosarcoma Study. Clin OrthopRelat Res. 1991;(270):8-14.

[10] Bloem JL, Kroon HM. Osseous lesions. Radiol Clin North Am 1993; 31: 61-78.

[11] Ozturk R, Bone and Soft Tissue Tumors. In: Atay T, ed. Orthopedics and Sport Medicine Guide for Researchers. Ankara; DermanMedical Publishing; 2015:635-704. DOİ: 10.4328/DERMAN.3774.

[12] Yamaguchi H, Minami A, Kaneda K, Isu K, Yamawaki S. Comparison of magnetic resonance imaging and computed tomography in the local assessment of osteosarcoma. Int Orthop. 1992;16(3):285-90. DOİ: 10.1007/BF00182713.

[13] Mankin Hj, Lange TA, Spanier SS. The hazards of biopsy in patients with malignant primary bone and soft tissue tumors. J Bone and Joint Surg Am 1982;64:1121-1127

[14] Hız M. Osteosarcoma, malignant fibrous histiocytoma – clinical radiology, pathology and treatment strategies. TOTBİ DDergisi 2014; 13:227-239 DOİ: 10.14292/totbid.dergisi.2014.25.

[15] Kaste SC, Pratt CB, Cain AM, Jones-Wallace DJ, Rao BN. Metastases detected at the time of diagnosis of primary pediatric extremity osteosarcoma at diagnosis: imaging features. Cancer. 1999;86(8):1602-8. DOİ: 10.1002/(sici)1097-0142(19991015)86:8<1602::aid-cncr31>3.0.co;2-r.

[16] Luetke A, Meyers PA, Lewis I, Juergens H. Osteosarcoma treatment - where do we stand? A state of the art review. Cancer Treat Rev.

2014;40(4):523-532. DOİ: 10.1016/j.ctrv.2013.11.006.

[17] Wittig JC, Bickels J, Priebat D, Jelinek J, Kellar-Graney K, Shmookler B, Malawer MM. Osteosarcoma: a multidisciplinary approach to diagnosis and treatment. Am Fam Physician. 2002;65(6):1123-1132.

[18] Philip T, Blay JY, Brunat-Mentigny M, Carrie C, Chauvot P, Farsi F, et al. French National Federation of Cancer (FNCLCC). Osteosarcoma. Br J Cancer. 2001;84 Suppl 2(Suppl 2):78-80. DOİ: 10.1054/bjoc.2000.1770.

[19] Harrison DJ, Geller DS, Gill JD, Lewis VO, Gorlick R. Current and future therapeutic approaches for osteosarcoma. Expert Rev Anticancer Ther. 2018;18(1):39-50. DOİ: 10.1080/14737140.2018.1413939.

[20] Meyers PA, Schwartz CL, Krailo M, Kleinerman ES, Betcher D, Bernstein ML, et al. Osteosarcoma: a randomized, prospective trial of the addition of ifosfamide and/or muramyl tripeptide to cisplatin, doxorubicin, and high-dose methotrexate. J Clin Oncol. 2005;23(9):2004-2011. DOİ: 10.1200/JCO.2005.06.031.

[21] Jaffe N, Carrasco H, Raymond K, Ayala A, Eftekhari F. Can cure in patients with osteosarcoma be achieved exclusively with chemotherapy and abrogation of surgery? Cancer. 2002;95(10):2202-10. DOİ: 10.1002/cncr.10944.

[22] Ando K, Heyman MF, Stresing V, Mori K, Rédini F, Heymann D. Current therapeutic strategies and noval approaches in osteosarcoma. Cancers (Basel) 2013;5(2):591-636. DOİ: 10.3390/cancers5020591.

[23] Capanna R, Scoccianti G, Frenos F, Vilardi A, Beltrami G, Campanacci DA. What was the survival of megaprostheses in lower limb reconstructions after tumor resections? Clin OrthopRelat Res. 2015;473(3):820-830. DOİ: 10.1007/s11999-014-3736-1.

[24] Campanacci M: Classic Osteosarcoma. İn: Campanacci M, ed. Bone and soft tissue tumors AuloGaggiEditore, Bologna 1990. P. 455-505.

[25] Bielack SS, Kempf-Bielack B, Delling G, Exner GU, Flege S, Helmke K. Prognostic factors in high-grade osteosarcoma of the extremities or trunk: an analysis of 1,702 patients treated on neoadjuvant cooperative osteosarcoma study group protocols. J Clin Oncol. 2002;20(3):776-790. DOİ: 10.1200/JCO.2002.20.3.776.

[26] Hagleitner MM, de Bont ES, te loo DM. Survival trends and long-term toxicity in pediatric patients with osteosarcoma. Sarcoma. 2012; 1-5. DOİ: 10.1155/2012/636405

[27] Marina NM, Smeland S, Bielack SS, Bernstein M, Jovic G, Krailo MD, et al. Comparison of MAPIE versus MAP in patients with a poor response to preoperative chemotherapy for newly diagnosed high-grade osteosarcoma (EURAMOS-1): an open-label, international, randomised controlled trial. Lancet Oncol. 2016;17(10):1396-1408. DOİ: 10.1016/S1470-2045(16)30214-5.

[28] Daw NC, Neel MD, Rao BN, Billups CA, Wu J, Jenkins JJ, et al. Frontline treatment of localized osteosarcoma without methotrexate: results of the St. Jude Children's Research Hospital OS99 trial. Cancer. 2011;117(12):2770-2778. DOİ: 10.1002/cncr.25715.

[29] Schwartz CL, Wexler LH, Krailo MD, Teot LA, Devidas M, Steinherz LJ, et al. Intensified Chemotherapy With Dexrazoxane Cardioprotection in Newly Diagnosed Nonmetastatic Osteosarcoma: A Report From the Children's Oncology Group. Pediatr Blood Cancer. 2016 Jan;63(1):54-61. doi: 10.1002/pbc.25753.

Section 2

Osteoarthritis

Chapter 6

Management of Early Osteoarthritis

Ahmed Mostafa Kotb Aziz

Abstract

Osteoarthritis (OA) is a chronic degenerative joint disease of dynamic pathology with multiple etiologies. It involves progressive process of softening, loss of articular cartilage, subchondral bone sclerosis, development of osteophytes, and cyst formation. OA usually contributes to decreased activity associated with aging, secondary to diminished function and pain, thus consequently impairing quality of life. It is well established that pain due to OA, swelling, or stiffness can make it difficult for individuals to perform simple daily living activities. Although OA is not curable, a variety of treatment modalities are available to improve symptoms. Main elements include pain management maneuvers, education, changing lifestyle physical activity (PA), and weight reduction in case of overweight. Although total joint arthroplasty (TJA) is considered a cost-effective treatment for people with OA, TJA should only be considered after failure of conservative treatments. Symptoms of OA are usually managed by either pharmachological or nonpharmachological protocols; joint replacement surgeries are considered in advanced cases. Analgesics remain the keystone of pharmacological treatment for OA symptoms, including paracetamol, topical and oral nonsteroidal anti-inflammatory drugs (NSAIDs), and opioids. However, benefits from paracetamol and opioids are minimal, and NSAIDs are not ideal for many patients because they have many side-effects. Intra-articular therapies such as corticosteroids are also commonly used, though usually with short-term benefits.

Keywords: early, osteoarthritis, hyaluronic acid, intraarticular

1. Introduction

Osteoarthritis (OA) is a chronic degenerative joint disease of dynamic pathology with multiple etiologies. It involves progressive process of softening, loss of articular cartilage, subchondral bone sclerosis, development of osteophytes, and cyst formation [1].

Knee OA is the most common arthritic disease among all joints; however, there is no available drug treatment today that hinders the progression of this disease process. There are many reasons for this, including the lack of understanding of what worsens the disease process and the heterogeneity of the patient population. There are considerable differences in the course of the disease [2].

The median age for diagnosis of Knee OA is 55 years, and usually people live about 30 years suffering the disease [3]. As there is no known curative treatment for OA till now, treatments aim at improving function as well as reducing pain.

IntechOpen

Systematic reviews (SR) are a useful research method to analyze the efficacy of knee OA treatments; however, most of these reviews have not discussed the long-term risks associated with various treatment modalities. The cause for that is most studies follow patients for short time periods. There are missing data in the literature owing to the fact that most of these studies are short-term studies, thus giving a false impression about the correct data concerning short-term improvement; especially, OA is a chronic condition needing long-term studies to correctly estimate the degree of pain improvement.

Approximately 30–65% of the risk of OA is genetically determined [4].

Obesity has long been known as a risk factor for knee OA [3]. A recent meta-analysis also showed that increased BMI added to the increased risks to radiographic and/or clinical OA picture [5].

OA usually contributes to decreased activity associated with aging, secondary to diminished function and pain, thus consequently impairing quality of life. It is well established that pain due to OA, swelling, or stiffness can make it difficult for individuals to perform simple daily living activities [6].

Researches on the role of special diets in OA have been evolving. High dietary fiber intake has been associated with lower risk of developing moderate to severe knee pain over time. Results from two prospective cohort studies also showed that increased total fiber intake was related to lower risk of symptomatic knee OA, but its association with radiographic knee OA is still not evident [7]. Another study found that increased soy milk intake was associated adversely with prevalence of radiographic knee osteophytes [8]. Finally, higher intake of Mediterranean diet was associated with lower prevalence of radiographic and clinical KOA [9].

The patient usually experiences knee pain and any three of the following to diagnose clinical OA of the knee: [1] tenderness on one or more knee compartments; [2] crepitus on active motion in at one or more knee compartments; [3] morning stiffness usually less than 30 minutes, according to WOMAC scale; [4] no warmth on knee examination; [3] age more than 50 years; or [5] osteophytes in one or more knee compartments [10].

Although OA is not curable, a variety of treatment modalities are available to improve symptoms. Main elements include pain management maneuvers, education, changing lifestyle physical activity (PA), and weight reduction in case of overweight. Although total joint arthroplasty (TJA) is considered a cost-effective treatment for people with OA, TJA should only be considered after failure of conservative treatments. Since OA is a chronic disease, a key element in the non-surgical management of knee and/or hip OA is self-management. Self-management interventions allow patients to improve their skills in taking care of themselves and to improve skills to navigate the health care system [11].

The shape of the bone may add to the risk of OA as had been described primarily in the hip joint. The association between OA and muscle strength may vary depending on the muscles and joints being studied. In an examination of anterior cruciate ligament (ACL) injured knees, high thigh muscle cross-sectional area and high muscle/fat ratio had a protective effect against KOA prevalence. Deformities of the knee are a strong predictor of knee OA disease progression [12].

Health education should be considered as a basic element of effective self-management interventions. Health education should include education about OA and its treatment options, exercise and pacing of PA, and weight reduction. This information should be tailored to the person's illness perception and educational capability. In addition, goal setting is a widely used behavioral change technique in many fields, especially in health care. Goal setting is associated with positive impact on behavior at both shorter and longer terms [13]. Behavioral monitoring of outcomes (e.g. amount of PA, weight and achievement of goals).

Symptoms of OA are usually managed by either pharmachological or nonpharmachological protocols; joint replacement surgeries are considered in advanced cases. Analgesics remain the keystone of pharmacological treatment for OA symptoms, including paracetamol, topical and oral nonsteroidal anti-inflammatory drugs (NSAIDs), and opioids. However, benefits from paracetamol and opioids are minimal, and NSAIDs are not ideal for many patients because they have many side-effects. Intra-articular therapies such as corticosteroids are also commonly used, though usually with short-term benefits. Pharmacological drugs include the following.

1.1 Colchicine

It is usually used for the treatment of pseudogout and gout. Colchicine is not recommended for treatment of OA nowadays. Synovial fluid in OA usually contains basic calcium phosphate (BCP) crystals especially hydroxyapatite crystals (detected in the cartilage of nearly all affected joints at the time of joint replacement surgeries). Positive correlations have been found between synovial fluid BCP crystal levels and radiographic severity of OA [14].

1.2 Hydroxychloroquine

Hydroxychloroquine has been used in in patients with inflammatory OA of hand joints with some suggested evidence of benefits, probably because it may have a role in treating rheumatoid arthritis (RA) synovitis and an acceptable safety profile. It has immunomodulatory effects and was considered to potentially treat OA due to Toll-like receptor (TLR) signaling inhibition, as TLRs are upregulated in OA cartilage and may have a role in cartilage breakdown *via* proinflammatory pathways [15].

A mixture of pharmacologic and nonpharmacologic therapies can manage OA symptoms as there is currently no available disease-modifying therapy till now, so treatment depends on symptomatic slow-acting drugs for OA (SYSADOAs) as an important category in the pharmacologic therapy tools for OA that have been demonstrated to alleviate the symptoms of functional impairment and pain, with some additional evidence of a disease-modifying effect on the long run [16]. The SYSADOAs class comprises different elements, including chondroitin, glucosamine, diacerein, and avocado soybean unsaponifiables (ASU), and there are some clinical data supporting their efficiency. Placebo-controlled trials of SYSADOAs treatment lasting up to 3 years in more than one Meta-analyses provide evidence that prescribing grade crystalline glucosamine sulfate (GS), chondroitin sulfate (CS), and diacerein has mild to moderate benefits in patients with OA [17].

Numerous meta-analyses and RCTs have been conducted to assess the efficacy and safety of Intra-articular hyaluronic acid (IAHA), with mixed results and conclusions support the fact that IAHA injection is considered a suitable alternative local treatment option providing symptomatic benefit without the systemic adverse effects that may be associated with IA corticosteroids. IAHA is considered to have a positive effect on pain and joint function. A meta-analysis comparing the effectiveness of pharmacological interventions for knee OA found that IAHA is considered an effective therapy. IAHA is also demonstrated to have a longer lasting effect on function and pain compared with IA corticosteroids, lasting up to 6 months [18].

Multiple courses of IAHA can cause long-term beneficial outcomes, including reduction in analgesics used and delay in the need for joint replacement surgeries [19] still found regarding the risk benefit of IAHA. However, controversy about lack of agreement among international guidelines regarding the use of IAHA for the management of symptomatic knee OA still exists [20].

The safety of IAHA has been evaluated in eight meta-analyses of RCTs comparing IAHA to IA placebo. However, a Cochrane review of 76 RCTs was unable to conclude a definitive report on the safety of HA due to limitations concerning sample size; however, no major safety issues were found, in addition, IAHA demonstrated similar efficacy to systemic forms of medical interventions, with more local reactions but fewer systemic adverse effects [21].

Evidence suggests that exercise is one of the core therapies for OA to improve function and pain. The degree of response varies according to the type of exercise (e.g. aerobic, strengthening, etc.). Little is known about the relative effeciency of different exercise forms [22].

The comparisons were seen between strengthening exercises and mixed exercises versus usual care. For pain, function, and performance, all types of exercise were significantly better than usual care. The largest effect was observed for aerobic and mind-body exercises for function and pain. Strengthening and flexibility exercises had a moderate score, whereas mixed exercise gave the minimum score for all outcomes and was significantly less effective than aerobic or mind-body exercise for pain. The ranking mainly corresponded to the magnitude of the score shown by each exercise. Aerobic exercises were the best-ranked for performance and pain, whereas mind-body was also the best-ranked for self-reported pain and function. Strengthening and flexibility/skill generally received mid-level rankings while mixed exercises were the least ranked exercise [23].

It is confirmed that exercise is still important for people suffering from hip and knee OA for outcomes of performance function, pain. In additon, it was found that mind-body and aerobic exercise have the largest score for improvements in function and pain; strengthening and flexibility exercises improve multiple outcomes to a varying degree [23]. Older age is a well-known risk factor for OA; women are more likely to develop hand, foot, and knee OA compared to men [4].

Varus thrust increased the odds of worsening medial bone marrow lesions (BMLs) and medial cartilage loss as well as the odds of incident medial BMLs of the knee among those with KOA and those with increased risk of Knee OA according to the Multicenter Osteoarthritis Study (MOST) [24].

It was found that aerobic exercises have similar effects to mind-body exercises for controlling pain. Mind-body exercise such as yoga and tai chi can be characterized as mild to moderate intensity exercise performed with an intentional awareness (mindfulness) on breathing and slow controlled movement [25]. Although the underlying mechanism is not clear, the effect of both mind-body and aerobic exercises may be related to the possibility that these exercises affect the altered central nervous system such as central pain sensitization, mood disorders, and sleep disturbance. Pain experience is the result of interactions between these central failure and peripheral pain mechanisms, as aerobic and mind-body exercise can influence both central and peripheral pain mechanisms. There is no satisfactory explanation for the poor effect of mixed exercise, particularly when considering that there are many domains of physical impairment in people with OA [23].

So far, NSAIDs, symptomatic slow-acting drugs for OA, analgesics, bone-acting agents, putative disease-modifying agents, and agents for intra-articular injection including HA and corticosteroids have been used as pharmacological agents for treating OA. However, it has been reported that these agents are not efficient against the main cause of OA, may cause some side effects, and are not adequate for the long-term management of OA. NSAIDs are the most commonly used drugs for the management of OA. They showed moderate improvement against OA pain; however, it is advised that NSAIDs be used intermittently and not advised for longer periods. NSAIDs can be classified as cyclooxygenase-2 selective agents and nonselective agents [26].

2. Putative disease-modifying agents

Putative disease-modifying drugs for OA like doxycycline, sprifermin, and cindunistat have not proved significant improvements of the joint so far although the clinical trials conducted to prove the effect of these drugs are still under trial [18].

3. Bone-acting agents

Bone-forming agents or antiresorptive agents like zoledronic acid, risedronate, strontium ranelate, calcitonin, and vitamin D are classified as bone-acting agents for the management of OA. They are bone-acting agents that showed some recorded effect in the turnover of subchondral bone, although these agents did not show a significant improvement in the structure of the joint [26].

4. Agents for intra-articular injection

Agents for intra-articular injection include HA and corticosteroids like triamcinolone, betamethasone, and methylprednisolone. Intra-articular injection of corticosteroids showed a greater beneficial effect. Furthermore, during follow-up periods of 3 and 6 months, intra-articular injection of HA showed a better therapeutic effect. Intra-articular injection of a combination of HA and corticosteroids showed a moderate beneficial effect on the pathological process of OA. However, for long-term pain control, intra-articular injection of HA did not show a significant improvement [26].

Use of nonpharmacological modalities (e.g. exercise) as a first-line management for knee OA is little to be compared with pharmacological modalities and usually associated with higher rates of surgical interventions. The results indicate that nonpharmacological agents such as exercise and weight reduction are effective in management of knee OA with minimal adverse side effects. Therefore, exercise and weight reduction should be advised as part of the treatment in most patients owing to their minimal side effects and cost effectiveness, as well as associated health benefits. It is important to specify resources and invest in supporting general practitioners and other primary health care providers to provide lifestyle interventions as a tool in managing knee OA [27].

Irrespective of a large body of evidence concerning the benefits of their use, opiates are used to manage pain associated with Knee OA. No studies fulfilled the inclusion criteria as the follow-up periods of these studies concerning safety were less than 6 months. A recent systematic review of chronic pain management found that there is insufficient evidence to support the effectiveness of long-term opioid therapy [28]. Opioids provide effective analgesia; however, benefits are usually encountered by frequent side effects such as nausea (30%), dizziness (20%), vomiting (13%), constipation (23%), and somnolence (18%) as well as the risk of addiction increases on chronic opioid use. The evidence on the safety and effectiveness of long-term opioid therapy for Knee OA cannot be evaluated. This is a concern and a limitation of the available evidence related to management of Knee OA. In the USA, there has been a significant increase in opioid prescriptions for patients suffering from knee OA, and opioids were prescribed to 15.9% of patients with knee OA [29].

Author details

Ahmed Mostafa Kotb Aziz
Ain Shams University, Cairo, Egypt

*Address all correspondence to: drakotb@live.com

References

[1] Charlesworth J et al. Osteoarthritis – A systematic review of long-term safety implications for osteoarthritis of the knee. BMC Musculoskeletal Disorders. 2019;**20**:151

[2] Karsdal MA, Michaelis M, Ladel C, et al. Disease-modifying treatments for osteoarthritis (DMOADs) of the knee and hip: Lessons learned from failures and opportunities for the future. Osteoarthritis and Cartilage. 2016;**24**:2013-2021

[3] Lane NE, Shidara K, Wise BL. Osteoarthritis year in review 2016: Clinical. Osteoarthritis and Cartilage. 2017;**25**:209-215

[4] Vina ER, Kwoh CK. Epidemiology of osteoarthritis: Literature update. Current Opinion in Rheumatology. 2018;**30**(2):160-167

[5] Jiang L, Xie X, Wang Y, et al. Body mass index and hand osteoarthritis susceptibility: An updated meta-analysis. International Journal of Rheumatic Diseases. 2016;**19**:1244-1254

[6] Marshall M, Watt FE, Vincent TL, et al. Hand osteoarthritis: Clinical phenotypes, molecular mechanisms and disease management. Nature Reviews Rheumatology. 2018;**14**:641-656

[7] Dai Z, Niu J, Zhang Y, et al. Dietary intake of fibre and risk of knee osteoarthritis in two US prospective cohorts. Annals of the Rheumatic Diseases. 2017;**76**:1411-1419

[8] Li H, Zeng C, Wei J, et al. Relationship between soy milk intake and radiographic knee joint space narrowing and osteophytes. Rheumatology International. 2016;**36**:1215-1222

[9] Veronese N, Stubbs B, Noale M, et al. Adherence to a Mediterranean diet is associated with lower prevalence of osteoarthritis: Data from the osteoarthritis initiative. American Journal of Clinical Nutrition. November 2016;**104**(5):1403-1409

[10] Clynes MA et al. Impact of osteoarthritis on activities of daily living: Does joint site matter? Aging Clinical and Experimental Research. 2019;**31**:1049-1056

[11] Pelle T et al. Development and evaluation of a tailored e-self-management intervention (dr. Bart app) for knee and/or hip osteoarthritis: Study protocol. BMC Musculoskeletal Disorders. 2019;**20**:398

[12] Jungmann PM, Baum T, Nevitt MC, et al. Degeneration in ACL injured knees with and without reconstruction in relation to muscle size and fat content-data from the osteoarthritis initiative. PLoS One. 2016;**11**:e0166865

[13] Epton T, Currie S, Armitage CJ. Unique effects of setting goals on behavior change: Systematic review and meta-analysis. Journal of Consulting and Clinical Psychology. 2017;**85**(12):1182-1198

[14] Ghouri A, Conaghan PG. Update on novel pharmacological therapies for osteoarthritis. Therapeutic Advances in Musculoskeletal Disease. 2019;**11**:1-11

[15] Sillat T, Barreto G, Clarijs P, et al. Tolllike receptors in human chondrocytes and osteoarthritic cartilage. Acta Orthopaedica. 2013;**84**:585-592

[16] Singh JA, Noorbaloochi S, MacDonald R, Maxwell LJ. Chondroitin for osteoarthritis. Cochrane Database of Systematic Reviews. 2015;**1**:CD005614

[17] Honvo G et al. Safety of symptomatic slow-acting drugs for

osteoarthritis: Outcomes of a systematic review and meta-analysis. Drugs & Aging. 2019;**36**(Suppl 1):S65-S99

[18] Pavelka K, Bruyere O, Cooper C, Kanis JA, Leeb BF, Maheu E, et al. Diacerein: Benefits, risks and place in the management of osteoarthritis. An opinion-based report from the ESCEO. Drugs & Aging. 2016;**33**(2):75-85

[19] Delbarre A, Amor B, Bardoulat I, Tetafort A, Pelletier-Fleury N. Do intra-articular hyaluronic acid injections delay total knee replacement in patients with osteoarthritis—A cox model analysis. PLoS One. 2017;**12**(11):e0187227

[20] Bannuru RR, Osani M, Vaysbrot EE, McAlindon TE. Comparative safety profile of hyaluronic acid products for knee osteoarthritis: A systematic review and network meta-analysis. Osteoarthritis and Cartilage. 2016;**24**(12):2022-2041

[21] Strand V, McIntyre LF, Beach WR, Miller LE, Block JE. Safety and efficacy of US-approved viscosupplements for knee osteoarthritis: A systematic review and meta-analysis of randomized, saline-controlled trials. Journal of Pain Research. 2015;**8**:217-228

[22] Bartels EM, Juhl CB, Christensen R, et al. Aquatic exercise for the treatment of knee and hip osteoarthritis. Cochrane Database of Systematic Reviews. 2016;**3**:CD005523

[23] Goh S-L et al. Relative efficacy of different exercises for pain, function, performance and quality of life in knee and hip osteoarthritis: Systematic review and network meta-analysis. Sports Medicine. 2019;**49**:743-761

[24] Wink AE, Gross KD, Brown CA, et al. Varus thrust during walking and the risk of incident and worsening medial tibiofemoral MRI lesions: The multicenter osteoarthritis study. Osteoarthritis and Cartilage. 2017;**25**:839-845

[25] Brosseau L, Taki J, Desjardins B, et al. The Ottawa panel clinical practice guidelines for the management of knee osteoarthritis. Part one: Introduction, and mind-body exercise programs. Clinical Rehabilitation. 2017;**31**(5):582-595

[26] Kang Y-H et al. Natural products as sources of novel drug candidates for the pharmacological management of osteoarthritis: A narrative review. Biomolecules & Therapeutics. 2019;**27**(6):503-513

[27] Gersing A, Schwaiger B, Nevitt M, et al. Is weight loss associated with less progression of changes in knee articular cartilage among obese and overweight patients as assessed with MR imaging over 48 months? Data from the osteoarthritis initiative. Radiología. 2017;**284**(2):508-520

[28] Volkow N, McLellan A. Opioid abuse in chronic pain-misconceptions and mitigation strategies. The New England Journal of Medicine. 2016;**374**(13):1253-1263

[29] DeMik D, Bedard N, Dowdle S, et al. Are we still prescribing opioids for osteoarthritis? The Journal of Arthroplasty. 2017;**S0883-5403**(17):30666

Chapter 7

Non-Surgical Regional Therapy for Osteoarthritis: An Update and Review of the Literature

Harold Wilson-Morkeh and Charles Mackworth-Young

Abstract

Osteoarthritis (OA) is the most common joint condition worldwide. It can lead to chronic debilitating symptoms that can be definitively managed with surgical techniques at times. More frequently however, either due to age, extent of disease or patient choice, non-surgical approaches are preferred. They include topical therapies such as thermotherapy, ultrasound, laser treatment, non-steroidal anti-inflammatory drugs (NSAIDs) and capsaicin cream. Injections are another technique often implemented. These consist of intra-articular (IA) corticosteroid or hyaluronan injections, trigger point injections and subcutaneous sodium salicylate. Acupuncture and various types of external support are also widely used. This chapter examines the latest evidence and summarises the role of the various regional treatments available for use in the management of OA.

Keywords: osteoarthritis, joint pain, regional therapy, topical therapy

1. Introduction

Osteoarthritis (OA) is the most common chronic joint condition in the world and affects nearly 9 million people in the United Kingdom alone [1]. It manifests clinically as localised joint pain, stiffness and occasionally swelling.

OA can occur as a primary idiopathic phenomenon with no prior causative trauma, although more frequent are cases of secondary OA appearing as a result of pre-existing joint damage [2]. This is often in the context of inflammatory arthropathy or previous injury. Risk factors for primary OA include advancing age, female sex, family history and obesity [1–3]. The disease can be restricted to a single joint or become more widespread, affecting multiple joints. In severe cases, it can progressively lead to significant deformity, loss of function and a reduced quality of life [1, 4].

Treatment has mainly focused on symptomatic relief from pain, physical approaches such as rehabilitation and physiotherapy, disease-modifying treatment (such as hydroxychloroquine) and surgery. Pain relief with systemic drugs has drawbacks. In particular, the use of non-steroidal anti-inflammatory drugs (NSAIDs) has been associated with significant adverse events including gastritis and increased risk of cardiovascular disease. In view of this, there has been increased interest in localised treatments for OA; specifically, therapies that are localised to the affected joint itself. These can be divided into topical treatment, such as anti-inflammatory gels, creams and thermotherapy, and more invasive local treatment including joint aspiration and intra-articular (IA) joint injection with corticosteroid and hyaluronans.

IntechOpen

2. Topical treatments

2.1 Thermotherapy

Thermotherapy refers to the application of either heat or cold (cryotherapy) to affected joints in an attempt to improve pain, stiffness and swelling.

Ice massage and the application of ice packs have both been studied in knee osteoarthritis [5–10]. It is likely that most of the observed effects of cryotherapy are related to the induction of local vasoconstriction. This leads to a reduction in blood flow, lower levels of local inflammation and reduced swelling. In one review [7], cryotherapy was found to reduce pain, stiffness and oedema. Regular ice massage, given five times a week, led to clinically significant effects on all three symptoms as well as function, strength and range of movement over a 2-week period [8]. However, these improvements were not replicated with less frequent applications (three times per week) [9]. There are no data to indicate a sustained effect of cold therapy on osteoarthritis as these studies looked only at a limited duration of therapy.

Common methods of superficial heat administration include the use of electrical heating pads, heat packs, towels or wax. Immersion in warm water or wax baths has also been shown to provide some subjective benefit. In some early trials, heat application failed to improve function or symptoms [8, 9]. In recent years, however, various studies have investigated different modalities of local heat therapy [10–13]. These include the application of heat packs [12], ultrasound [11, 13] and diathermy. The application of local heat packs has been found to provide short-lived alleviation of pain [12, 14], and in particular, wet heat (involving liquids) has been found to be better than dry heat [15] for symptomatic improvement.

In one study [12] 18 patients were randomised into two groups that received differing therapy over a course of 12 weeks. One was treated with application of steam generating heat sheets for 6 hours each day, and the other performed a daily quadriceps strengthening exercise regime. At the end of the study, patients in the heat-treated group reported statistically significant improvements in their symptoms and objective "Up and Go" times (a measure of function). The mechanism of heat therapy in osteoarthritis is unclear, although ex vivo studies of cartilage [15, 16] have indicated that elevating the temperature of chondrocytes may increase their metabolism and the production of proteoglycans that are major components of cartilage in combination with collagen. This, in part, may be secondary to increased blood flow to the chondrocytes.

On the whole, the available data suggest that thermotherapy may be useful as an adjunct in the treatment of osteoarthritis, although long-term benefits have not been established, and there are no robust clinical trials evaluating its efficacy.

2.2 Local ultrasound therapy

The role of ultrasound (US) in diagnosis of musculoskeletal problems is well established. Its popularity is in large part due to the low cost and non-invasive nature of the modality. In recent years, there has been growing interest in its application for therapeutic purposes [13, 17–19]. In theory, direct treatment with US leads to local heating of the tissue at depths not achieved by applying heat packs. There are two main techniques utilised: continuous US which leads to a rise in temperature of the treated tissues, enhancing fibrous tissue extensibility [20] and promoting capillary permeability [21] and pulsed wave treatment which harnesses nonthermal effects and is beneficial for cartilage health [18].

In vitro and animal studies [17, 18] have suggested that pulsed wave US can increase collagen production and reduce expression of membrane metalloproteinase, suggesting a protective role. However, this has failed to translate to long-term clinical benefit: randomised controlled studies [13, 19] comparing continuous, pulsed and sham US on knee osteoarthritis symptoms have shown no significant difference in pain scores nor function. In general, the safety of US has been established, and anecdotal trends have been observed, but evidence is scarce for any significant therapeutic advantage [13, 19].

2.3 Laser therapy

Laser beam therapy directs intense light to treated tissue. Two types of laser therapy have been trialled in osteoarthritis: low-level and high-intensity. Low-level laser therapy (LLLT) uses red and infrared light wavelengths, whilst high-intensity laser therapy confers higher wavelengths of radiation for deeper tissue penetration. LLLT produces a photochemical rather than thermal response and has been found to reduce pain by modulating the local inflammatory process at a cellular level [22]. This involves the increased production of reactive oxygen species (ROS) and enables transcription of cellular components such as nuclear factor kappa-light-chain-enhancer of activated B cells (NF-κB) that help modulate cell proliferation and growth (**Figure 1**).

In one rat model of osteoarthritis, laser therapy caused a reduction in neutrophil migration, oxidative stress, altered levels of cyclooxygenase-2 and other pro-inflammatory mediators [24]. Another demonstrated that LLLT stimulates tissue repair and reduces the rate of extracellular matrix degradation [25]. There is also some evidence that LLLT promotes fibroblast proliferation, collagen synthesis and bone regeneration [26–31]. In a rabbit model of osteoarthritis, 6 weeks of treatment with laser therapy not only resulted in less pain but also histological evidence of reduced inflammation and cartilage damage [32].

This suggests that LLLT could have disease-modifying effects as well as symptomatic benefits, although the results of early clinical trials have been mixed thus far [33].

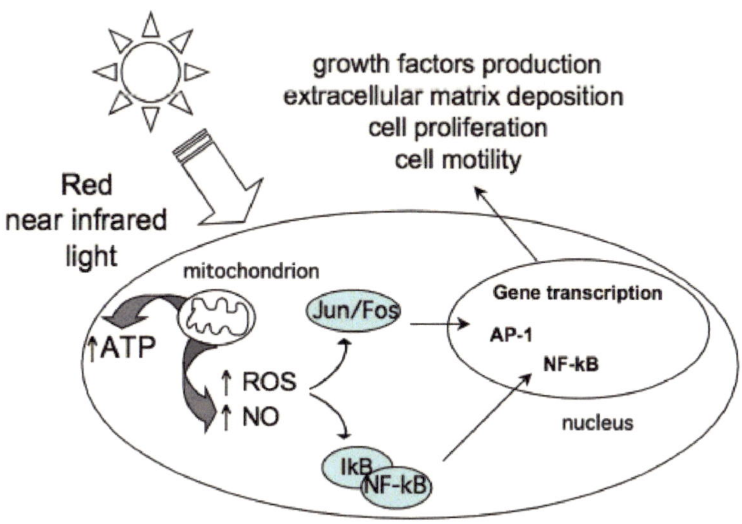

Figure 1.
Mechanisms of low-level light therapy (reproduced from Ref. [23]). Abbreviations: ATP, adenosine triphosphate; ROS, reactive oxygen species; NO, nitric oxide; Jun/Fos, Jun and Fos protein subunits; IκB, inhibitor of kappa B; NF-κB, nuclear factor kappa-light-chain-enhancer of activated B cells; AP-1, activator protein-1.

Recent studies have tended to be more positive with those treated with laser therapy and exercise faring better than those treated with exercise alone in terms of pain measurements as well as function [34, 35]. These studies suggest that LLLT in combination with standard physiotherapy could provide advantages over standard therapy, and it shows potential as a non-invasive, safe and cost-efficient treatment modality [36]. Once again, however, evidence is lacking regarding long-term effects and whether the cellular effects seen modify disease progression.

2.4 Topical non-steroidal anti-inflammatory drugs

The mechanism of action of non-steroidal anti-inflammatory drugs is well-known. They inhibit the action of cyclooxygenases (COXs) responsible for the synthesis of prostaglandins (PGs), which are recognised mediators of inflammation [37]. Locally this reduces pain, swelling and heat. There is a large body of evidence in animal models of NSAIDs also providing central analgesic actions, with mechanisms involving spinal regulation of COXs and PGs as well as the induction of endogenous opioid peptides and blockade of serotonin release [38].

It is clear to see, therefore, why systemic NSAIDs have long been used in management of osteoarthritis. However, significant side effects including gastritis, renal impairment and increased risk of cardiovascular disease has meant that their long-term use has been limited. This has led to the promotion of topical NSAID use, theoretically providing local analgesic and anti-inflammatory benefits without the undesirable systemic adverse effects.

There are many types of topical NSAID. Preparations containing diclofenac, ibuprofen, piroxicam, ketoprofen or felbinac as the active ingredient all exist. Some include a penetration enhancer such as menthol or dimethyl sulfoxide (DMSO), whilst gels and sprays tend to be more penetrative than cream preparations. Once applied, a topical NSAID is absorbed by the underlying tissue or enters the local blood stream. Studies have shown that the absorption of NSAIDs into the underlying tissue gives rise to therapeutic local concentrations of the drug without significant systemic absorption [39, 40]. An estimated 3–7% of the applied dose is thought to be absorbed systemically [39] with plasma concentrations approximately 5% of those achieved with oral administration [39].

The skin acts as a reservoir from which the drug disseminates to the deeper tissue. Peak concentrations in the skin are achieved 2 hours after application with a further spike approximately 19 hours later, likely secondary to systemic absorption. Further proof of their local action is the absence of analgesic effect at joints distant to the point of application [41].

There have been many studies looking into the efficacy of topical NSAIDs in treating osteoarthritis [42–48]. On the whole, these have found topical NSAIDs to be superior to placebo in the treatment of chronic pain. Most of the initial studies found no benefit beyond 2 weeks of treatment [42–48], but larger randomised controlled trials demonstrated long-term benefit for up to 3 months when compared to placebo [49, 50].

When compared to oral NSAID use, the results have been variable. A meta-analysis in 2006 [48] found that topical NSAIDs were less effective than systemic NSAIDs. Since then, however, there have been several studies showing comparable effectiveness. Two studies comparing oral diclofenac with a topical preparation of the drug [51, 52] found no difference in pain scores or physical function. Furthermore, those in the topical treatment arm had a much lower incidence of severe gastrointestinal side effects, deranged liver function tests and abnormal creatinine clearance [51, 52]. These results were replicated in another study comparing oral and topical treatment with ibuprofen for knee osteoarthritis [50].

On the whole, topical NSAID use is associated with fewer systemic adverse events [42, 46, 51, 52] than oral preparations. The main side effect associated with topical NSAID use is local skin irritation, which has been reported in up to 39.3% of patients [53]. However, these skin reactions occur in equal measure with placebo gel application indicating that they may not be related to the active drug itself [46]. Other studies also suggest that skin reactions may be more common with solutions containing DMSO than diclofenac sodium gel (DSG) [44]. There is some contradictory evidence regarding their safety in older patients as some studies have found the rate of gastrointestinal side effects in the over 50s to be as high as 15% [53].

Overall, the data suggest that topical NSAIDs may be considered as first-line therapy for osteoarthritis as they are efficacious and associated with fewer adverse events. As with oral use, however, there should still be caution about their long-term application in the elderly as these patients are known to be more prone to adverse events.

2.5 Other topical treatments

Topical capsaicin cream has been used to treat a multitude of different painful conditions including osteoarthritis, inflammatory arthritis and neuropathic pain. Derived from chilli peppers, capsaicin is a lipophilic alkaloid that acts as a local irritant. It activates local pain receptors (c-nociceptors) leading to the release of substance P [54]. This in turn causes local irritation in the initial phase of treatment. With repeated use, however, levels of substance P are depleted, leading to desensitisation of the pain fibres and hypoalgesia [55].

In clinical practice, capsaicin is more effective than placebo for the treatment of chronic pain but compares less favourably with other treatments. In a meta-analysis comparing capsaicin with plaster for instance, capsaicin was found to be only marginally effective [56]. Other drawbacks include the need to use the cream four times a day for maximum benefit, as well as the local irritation and burning sensation when the cream is applied (occurring in up to 40% of patients) [57, 58]. These problems cause 10% of patients to discontinue treatment [56]. In view of this, topical capsaicin should be used in conjunction with more traditional treatments.

Other topical treatments include the use of salicylate or nicotine esters, which can be classed as local counterirritants and rubefacients, and lidocaine patches. Rubefacients cause localised vasodilatation and reddening of the skin that result in a local sensation of warmth, which often palliates pain. Irritation of the sensory nerve endings in underlying muscle and tissue is a by-product of their application and thought to modify pain pathways [59], but their main action is regional skin irritation.

The available evidence does not support their use for acute injuries or for chronic conditions such as osteoarthritis, though they are relatively well tolerated in the short term [60]. When compared to topical NSAIDs, counterirritants performed poorly [60]. This has led to numerous recommendations advising the discontinuation of routine rubefacient prescriptions in England, with patients signposted to alternative, more efficacious local treatments [61].

Lidocaine patches are not currently licensed for use in osteoarthritis in the United Kingdom, instead being more commonly utilised in the context of post-herpetic neuralgia. There is some anecdotal evidence for their efficacy in OA, however [62]. Lidocaine forms cations following ionisation with hydrogen ions and reversibly inhibits voltage-gated sodium channels on the internal surface of neuronal surface membranes when bound [63]. This prevents an influx of sodium cations (**Figure 2**) which in turn leads to a failure of nerve depolarisation resulting in the diminished pain signalling that has been observed in some clinical trials.

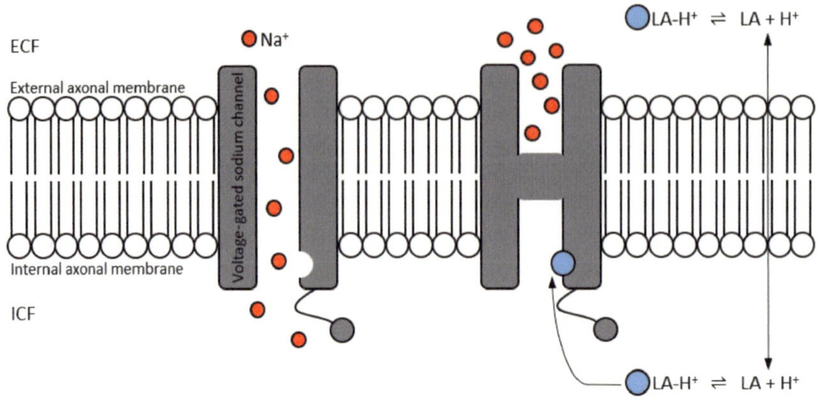

Figure 2.
The effect of lidocaine on a voltage-gated sodium channel. Abbreviations: LA, lidocaine; Na, sodium; H, hydrogen, ECF, extracellular fluid, ICF, intracellular fluid.

One open-label multicentre study investigated the effect of application of lidocaine to the area of maximal OA pain in OA of the knee [62]. A 5% lidocaine patch was applied for 12 hours at the same time each day for a period of 2 weeks with significant improvement in pain and functional scores when this treatment was used as an adjunct to more conventional systemic analgesia. Furthermore, there were minimal adverse effects seen, and the treatment was well tolerated in the patient cohort.

Clearly, randomised control trials are required to support the anecdotal data, as a sustained benefit has yet to be proven. It should also be noted that the symptomatic improvement observed was related to the use of a lidocaine patch as an adjunct to therapy, rather than a lone therapeutic agent in the management of OA. As in the case of capsaicin or rubefacients, lidocaine acts as a painkiller but has no disease-modifying capacity.

3. Local injections

3.1 Intra-articular corticosteroids

Intra-articular corticosteroid injections are frequently used to treat osteoarthritis. They work locally via anti-inflammatory effects, inhibiting the inflammatory cascade predominantly through the glucocorticoid receptor (GR) on both genomic and non-genomic levels (**Figure 3**). The genomic pathway largely comprises GR binding leading to the recruitment of complexes that influence the activity of RNA polymerase II. This affects gene transcription and repression. The GR also directly binds subunits of transcription factors such as NF-κB and activator protein-1 (AP-1), interfering with their activation and inhibiting the production of pro-inflammatory cytokines.

The non-genomic pathway is set in motion within seconds of GR binding. Various signalling cascades are activated such as those that inhibit phospholipase A2 activation and subsequent arachidonic acid release. These result in a downregulation of cyclic endoperoxides that are key components of the inflammatory response [65].

Local injection avoids many of the systemic problems associated with oral corticosteroid use and allows delivery of high doses to the affected tissue. Response to IA injection, however, does not appear to be dependent on inflammation within the affected joint itself [66]. Additional studies looking at whether inflammation detected on ultrasound predicted clinical response found that those without inflammatory

	GENOMIC	NON-GENOMIC
MEDIATOR	GR (cytosolic)	GR (cytosolic or membrane-bound)
MAIN TARGETS	RNA Polymerase II NF-κB (p65 subunit) AP-1 (Jun subunit)	PI3K AKT MAPKs
LATENCY	Hours	Seconds to minutes
RESPONSE	Activation of gene transcription and repression	Inhibition of phospholipase A2 Phosphorylation of annexin 1 Impaired release of arachidonic acid

Figure 3.
Summary of the glucocorticoid signalling pathways (reproduced from Ref. [64]). Abbreviations: GR, glucocorticoid receptor; NF-κB, nuclear factor kappa-light-chain-enhancer of activated B cells; AP-1, activator protein-1; PI3K, phosphoinositide 3-kinase; AKT, RAC-alpha serine/threonine-protein kinase; MAPKs, mitogen-activated protein kinases.

change fared better in response to IA injection than those with evidence of inflammation. Furthermore, the presence of synovial thickening, synovial fluid volume and white cell count did not predict better response to IA injection [66, 67]. In knee OA, joint aspiration prior to IA injection appears to provide greater symptomatic benefit [67]. This is partly due to anatomical confirmation on prior aspiration and concentrated drug delivery due to a lower volume of overall synovial fluid [68].

Commonly, IA injections are diluted with local anaesthetic to provide immediate relief, ensure accurate drug delivery and allow even dispersal of the drug within the joint due to the larger volume [69]. Frequently used corticosteroids in IA injections include hydrocortisone acetate (HCA), methylprednisolone acetate (MPA) and triamcinolone acetonide (TCA). These vary in solubility with the HCA being the most soluble of these three and TCA the least soluble. Less soluble preparations are longer acting and theoretically provide more long-term relief.

This effect is not always observed in clinical practice, however. In one randomised control trial comparing MPA (more soluble and shorter acting) and TCA in knee osteoarthritis, greater improvement in pain scores was found in the TCA group at 3 weeks than in MPA, although there was no difference between the two groups at 8 weeks [70]. There was also no significant difference in functional scores [70].

Further studies have investigated whether IA steroid injections provide symptomatic or functional benefit in knee osteoarthritis [66, 67, 71, 72]. These demonstrated short-term improvement in pain generally up to 4 weeks, though a small proportion of patients reported benefit to 6 weeks. Conversely, no improvement in function was seen when compared to placebo, and follow-up beyond 6 weeks did not reveal longer-lasting benefits. These results were further corroborated in a Cochrane systematic review [73]. This suggests IA steroid injections should be used as a short-term bridging treatment to resolve acute painful flares pending further intervention such as physiotherapy or surgery. Similar trials observing IA injections in the hip echo the results of those studies focusing on the knee: patients gained rapid and short-lived pain relief following injection, but these benefits were not maintained beyond 1 month [74, 75].

Other studies, focused specifically on another joint commonly affected by osteoarthritis, the first carpometacarpal (CMC) joint, uncovered more variable results related to long-term relief. In one study of 40 patients, no benefit was observed between IA steroid injection when compared to placebo [76]. Unsurprisingly, patients less likely to have sustained long-term benefits had more significant radiographic appearances (increased number of osteophytes and advanced joint space narrowing) [77]. In patients with less advanced disease, IA first CMC joint injection could provide symptomatic relief for up to 18 months following injection and splinting [77].

Although IA injections avoid the potentially toxic side effects of systemic steroids, they are not without risks themselves. All patients undergoing IA injection should be consented for the risk of infection, although this is a rare event (incidence reported between 1 in 3000 and 1 in 50,000) [78] and may be clinically difficult to differentiate from an injection-induced crystal arthritis which can occur in 2–6% of patients [67, 71]. In general, septic arthritis following IA injection occurs 3–4 days post procedure. There is a risk of lipoatrophy at the site of injection (estimated 0.6% of patients) [79], although this can be reduced by using shorter-acting preparations. Other serious local adverse events include tendon rupture, muscle wasting and local depigmentation. These risks can be minimised by performing image-guided injections where possible.

Systemic adverse events are rare with local corticosteroid injections, but as there is evidence for systemic absorption, they do still occur [80]. The most common is flushing which occurs in up to 40% of patients [81]. There have been reported incidents of unstable diabetic glycaemic control postinjection but this tends to be minor and usually settles [82]. Studies looking at the endocrine axis in patients who had received IA steroid injections found that serum cortisol dipped 24–48 hours after IA injection and took up to 4 weeks to return to baseline [80]. Major complications, such as steroid-induced osteoporosis, have not been observed, however [82].

Studies in animals have suggested that IA steroids can induce chondrocyte degeneration [83], but prospective clinical trials where patients received regular IA injections have failed to demonstrate an increased rate of cartilage loss [84]. There are also limited data to support a significant increased risk of osteonecrosis in injected joints. Nevertheless, repeated IA injections offer no long-term benefit [73] and should generally be avoided except for rapid pain relief in the short term in the absence of superior alternatives.

3.2 Intra-articular hyaluronic acid/hyaluronan

Hyaluronic acid (HA), also known as hyaluronan, is a large glycosaminoglycan molecule found in synovial and cartilage extracellular matrix (ECM). It is produced by synoviocytes, chondrocytes and fibroblasts and functions as both a lubricant and a means to maintain hydration within the joint [85]. Studies have shown that osteoarthritic joints have decreased hyaluronan content in the synovial fluid [86] and therefore IA injection with a synthetic analogue was a method developed to restore the function in degenerative joints.

Chondroprotection is the most frequent mechanism proposed in favour of the use of IA-HA [87]. This term specifically refers to the reduction of chondrocyte apoptosis as well as an increase in chondrocyte proliferation that occurs when HA binds to CD44 receptors. This results in inhibition of the well-known pro-inflammatory cytokine interleukin (IL)-1β through induction of mitogen-activated protein kinase phosphatase (MKP)-1 [88].

Synthetic preparations of HA closely mimic endogenous molecules. Later preparations contain cross-linked hyaluronan in order to achieve greater elasticity and viscosity. In theory, this confers greater intra-articular durability of the solution. Preparations with a higher molecular weight also seem to be more beneficial than those with a lower weight [89]. This may be related to the difference in volume required for injection, the number of injections required and the intra-articular durability of the solution.

Multiple studies have been conducted investigating the efficacy of IA injections of hyaluronans in osteoarthritis, mostly affecting the knee, and the evidence to support their use has been mixed. In general, HA appears to be better than placebo in improving pain scores, function and patient global assessment in the context of knee osteoarthritis [90]. The greatest clinical benefit is achieved at week 5–13 after a course of treatment of several injections. However, one of the drawbacks of the available data is the wide variability in trial design, frequency of injections and molecular weight of the administered synthetic product. Additionally, in hip OA, HA injections were not superior to placebo or corticosteroid injections in reducing pain or improving function [91]. There were similar findings in studies looking at OA of the hand [92].

Though HA is relatively safe, its use is restricted by the relatively high cost of the treatment [87]. It is generally reserved for knee osteoarthritis and, like corticosteroid, is offered either as a holding measure until more definitive treatment can be undertaken (e.g. surgery) or in patients for whom such treatment is inappropriate.

3.3 Subcutaneous and soft tissue injections

Trigger points are localised areas of tenderness and thickening in the soft tissues. They are typically located proximal to an inflamed or painful joint such as the rectus femoris in patients with knee OA and paraspinal regions in the cervical and lumbar spine [93]. They have also been described as interstitial fibrositis, myofasciitis and myofascial trigger points [94–96]. The aetiology and pathogenesis of trigger points are unknown.

Trigger point injections (TPI) have been used as a way of alleviating pain and discomfort associated with these areas of thickening. This can be via direct injection of medication (e.g. local anaesthetic and/or corticosteroid) into the point of tenderness or indirect needling of the soft tissue in that area. The trigger point is identified as the maximal area of tenderness in the muscle and is usually isolated by the thumb and forefinger to prevent movement in the underlying muscle. A small sterile needle is then introduced into the area, and the substance is injected directly within. Alternatively, a dry needle approach (without medication) can be used. If the injection is performed correctly, there is typically an initial acute worsening of pain associated with muscle spasm [97].

A systematic review of TPI in the management of chronic musculoskeletal pain revealed an improvement in symptoms when used exclusively [98]. This was irrespective of the injectant used [98]. The addition of a local anaesthetic, however, has been found to reduce the pain and irritation that is temporarily caused by the procedure [96].

There are limited data on the efficacy of TPI in the treatment of osteoarthritis. One study found that TPI in conjunction with IA corticosteroid was more effective than IA injection alone evidenced in both pain and functional scores [99]. Other studies have looked at TPI as sole treatment for OA, but this does not reflect clinical practice. Overall, TPI is safe and can be used as additional therapy in OA, though consideration should be made on a case-by-case basis.

Medication used in TPI includes local anaesthetic, corticosteroids, anti-inflammatories such as acetylsalicylate and ketorolac, as well as saline and water [96, 100–104]. There have also been several studies looking at the use of subcutaneous salicylate therapy for OA. In one trial 40 patients with OA of the first CMC joint [105] were randomised to receive either sham injection or subcutaneous injection with salicylate into trigger points. Patients were assessed blindly at 3, 7 and 13 weeks. Pain scores were significantly lower in those treated with salicylate than with sham injections [105].

The mechanism of action of subcutaneous salicylate injections is unclear, particularly as the site of injection is not within the affected joint. One theory is that salicylate may alter central sensitisation, and this is supported by the immediate relief patients report following injection. An alternative hypothesis is that the local effect of salicylate modifies the neurogenic control of inflammation, which may be abnormal in diseases that affect musculoskeletal structures such as OA [106, 107]. Changes in the expression and transport of neurogenic peptides may be induced by the local irritant effect of salicylate [108]. Systemic anti-inflammatory effects are unlikely, since the benefits are generally not observed in distant sites [105].

There is a degree of overlap between TPI and acupuncture in that the injection sites are standard acupuncture locations. Acupuncture involves the insertion of fine filiform needles at or near the tender anatomical site or sometimes at distant acupuncture "points". In a variation of this, the needles are sometimes stimulated electronically or with heat. Patients typically receive six or more sessions for a complete course of treatment. A systematic review of 393 patients with OA found acupuncture significantly improved pain but not function when compared to sham acupuncture [109–116]. In addition, results were no better than standard treatment with physiotherapy or being on a waiting list to receive acupuncture [109, 112]. There was also no additional benefit seen when using acupuncture as an adjunct to standard therapy with exercise and advice [115]. Moreover, there is little evidence for long-term benefit following acupuncture treatment, as symptomatic improvements tend to last up to 12 weeks only [109, 112]. Acupuncture is relatively safe, however, with minimal risks of serious side effects [113–116].

4. Orthoses

Osteoarthritic joints may be reinforced by various forms of external support known as orthoses. These applied devices modify the structural and functional characteristics of the neuromusculoskeletal system. Benefit can be obtained by adjusting alignment, reducing stress or load, providing shock absorption or simply resting the joint.

Orthoses such as braces, splints and elasticated sleeves are frequently used in OA of the hand and knee. Thumb and wrist splints are employed in hand OA, whilst knee sleeves and unloading braces can be useful adjuncts in knee OA. Medial patellar strapping can be specifically helpful for patellar maltracking [117]. Shoe insoles may be of benefit in OA affecting the ankle and knee and can sometimes alleviate symptoms caused by OA of the hip. Insoles can be differentiated into cushioned or neutral subtypes, which have shock-absorbing properties, and wedged insoles, which offset varus or valgus deformities as well as modulate mechanical stress.

For OA of the knee and ankle, the main purpose of orthoses and insoles is to support a joint that is unstable and to help correct alignment [118]. They can modify load bearing, contribute to pain reduction and improve physical function. There is also some evidence that they can improve proprioception [119] and they may slow disease progression [120]. They are especially useful for mild or moderate uni-compartmental knee OA where there may be varying degrees of instability and malalignment [121, 122].

Unloading knee braces are designed to reduce the load transmitted to the affected compartment by applying an external valgus or varus force. Symptomatic relief is achieved by stabilising the joint, increasing joint opening and reducing local muscle contraction [120]. One study [123] demonstrated that patients with medial compartment knee OA treated with unloading knee braces had better functional and symptomatic outcomes at 6 months. These results were not replicated in other studies [124] although there is evidence they can improve quadricep strength and gait symmetry [125].

The main disadvantage of these braces is poor tolerability due to the weight and heat of the device. In one study, 41% of patients complained of skin irritation [126], and up to 20% of patients discontinue use within 6 months [127]. Overall, there is limited evidence that braces or insoles provide an additional beneficial effect for knee OA when compared with medical treatment alone [128].

On the other hand, splinting of the thumb CMC joint has been found to be helpful in improving function and pain [129]. CMC joint OA contributes more to pain and disability than interphalangeal joint OA [130], and thus splinting of the CMC joint is logical. In a systematic review in 2010, CMC splinting was found to improve function and grip strength [129]. Further RCT data has corroborated this finding and demonstrated sustained benefit at 12 months [131]. However, these splints are inevitably somewhat cumbersome to wear and inhibit many day-to-day manual functions.

In general, splinting might be useful for symptomatic relief and may even improve function with prolonged use in appropriately selected patients.

5. Mesenchymal stem cells

The next frontier in local osteoarthritis management is likely to involve the use of mesenchymal stem cells (MSCs). These pluripotent cells have the capacity to differentiate into a variety of cell types, including chondrocytes, making their potential use in osteoarthritis a highly attractive prospect [132].

MSCs can undergo chondrogenesis and have been combined with a number of materials that support this differentiation, including the aforementioned polymer HA [133]. Neocartilage formation, hypertrophy and matrix calcification, as is seen in the terminal differentiation of hypertrophic chondrocytes in the growth plate, have been observed in vitro [134] and in mice [135] resulting in the efficient formation of bone. There are various hypotheses as to how this might occur. They include the inhibition of apoptosis [136] and subsequent immunomodulation [137] both of which are currently being tested in murine models of OA.

Clearly, translation to human studies is required before MSCs become a viable clinical option in the local treatment of OA, but there is understandable optimism that this therapy may herald a long-term solution to slowing the rate of articular cartilaginous degeneration and subchondral bone remodelling.

6. Conclusion

There are numerous local treatments for osteoarthritis. The majority of local therapies are safe and avoid any significant systemic adverse effects. They mostly provide symptomatic relief. In many cases this is of undoubted value to individual patients, particularly during the inflammatory phase of OA. In some cases there may be a useful placebo effect. In general, these therapies should be used as adjuncts to physiotherapy and systemic analgesia which remain the mainstay of conservative OA management. The choice of local therapy in an individual patient should be guided by the severity of disease, local experience and patient preference.

Some of these treatments, for instance, IA injections and orthoses, are well established and have been used in clinical practice for many decades. Other more novel approaches have been developed such as local laser therapy and subcutaneous sodium salicylate injections. However, for all the therapies described in this chapter, there are only limited data to demonstrate long-term benefit. Further studies are required to establish their lasting value. In the meantime these treatments remain valuable as temporary measures for many patients, particularly those with flares of symptoms or who are awaiting more definitive treatment.

Author details

Harold Wilson-Morkeh[1] and Charles Mackworth-Young[2*]

1 Department of Rheumatology, Hammersmith Hospital, Imperial College Healthcare NHS Trust, London, United Kingdom

2 Department of Rheumatology, Charing Cross Hospital, Imperial College Healthcare NHS Trust, London, United Kingdom

*Address all correspondence to: c.mackworth-young@imperial.ac.uk

References

[1] Neogi T. The epidemiology and impact of pain in osteoarthritis. Osteoarthritis and Cartilage. 2013;**21**(9):1145-1153

[2] Haq I, Murphy E, Dacre J. Osteoarthritis. Postgraduate Medical Journal. 2003;**79**(933):377-383

[3] Zhang Y, Jordan JM. Epidemiology of osteoarthritis. Clinics in Geriatric Medicine. 2010;**26**(3):355-369

[4] Zhang Y, Niu J, Kelly-Hayes M, Chaisson CE, Aliabadi P, Felson DT. Prevalence of symptomatic hand osteoarthritis and its impact on functional status among the elderly: The Framingham Study. American Journal of Epidemiology. 2002;**156**(11):1021-1027

[5] Cameron MH. Physical Agents in Rehabilitation. From Research to Practice. Philadelphia: WB Saunders Company; 1999

[6] Arthritis Foundation. Osteoarthritis. 2017. Available from: https://www.arthritis.org/about-arthritis/types/osteoarthritis

[7] Brosseau L, Yonge KA, Robinson V, Marchand S, Judd M, Wells G, et al. Thermotherapy for treatment of osteoarthritis. Cochrane Database of Systematic Reviews. 2003;**4**:CD004522

[8] Yurtkuran M, Kocagil T. TENS, electroacupuncture and ice massage: Comparison of treatment for osteoarthritis of the knee. American Journal of Acupuncture. 1999;**27**(3-4):133-140

[9] Clarke GR, Willis LA, Stenner L, Nichols PJR. Evaluation of physiotherapy in the treatment of osteoarthrosis of the knee. Rheumatology and Rehabilitation. 1974;**13**(4):190-197

[10] Hecht PJ, Bachmann S, Booth RE Jr, Rothman RH. Effects of thermal therapy on rehabilitation after total knee arthroplasty: A prospective randomized study. Clinical Orthopaedics and Related Research. 1983;**178**:198-201

[11] Boyaci A, Tutoglu A, Boyaci N, Aridici R, Koca I. Comparison of the efficacy of ketoprofe phonophoresis, ultrasound and short-wave diathermy in knee osteoarthritis. Rheumatology International. 2013;**33**(11):2811-2818

[12] Ochiai S, Watanabe A, Oda H, Ikeda H. Effectiveness of thermotherapy using a heat and steam generating sheet for cartilage in Knee osteoarthritis. Journal of Physical Therapy Science. 2014;**26**:281-284

[13] Cakir S, Hepguler S, Ozturk C, Korkmaz M, Iseleten B, Atamaz FC. Efficacy of therapeutic ultrasound for the management of knee osteoarthritis: a randomised controlled and double-blind study. American Journal of Physical Medicine & Rehabilitation. 2014;**93**(5):405-412

[14] Michlovitz S, Hun L, Erasala GN. Continuous low-level heat wrap therapy is effective for treating wrist pain. Archives of Physical Medicine and Rehabilitation. 2004;**85**:1409-1416

[15] Petrofsky JS, Bains G, Raju C. The effect of moisture content of a local heat source on the blood flow response of the skin. Archives of Dermatological Research. 2009;**301**:581-585

[16] Brand HS, De Koning MH, Van Kampen GP. Effect of temperature on the metabolism of proteoglycans in explants of bovine articular cartilage. Connective Tissue Research. 1991;**26**:87-100

[17] Li X, Li J, Cheng K, Lin Q, Wang D, Zhang H, et al. Effect of low-intensity pulsed ultrasound on MMP-13 and MAPKs signaling pathway in rabbit

knee osteoarthritis. Cell Biochemistry and Biophysics. 2011;**61**(2):427-434

[18] Naito K, Watari T, Muta T, Furuhata A, Iwase H, Igarashi M, et al. Low-intensity pulsed ultrasound (LIPUS) increases the articular cartilage type II collagen in a rat osteoarthritis model. Journal of Orthopaedic Research. 2010;**28**(3):361-369

[19] Ulus Y, Tander B, Akyol Y, Durmus D, Buyukakıncak O, Gul U, et al. Therapeutic ultrasound versus sham ultrasound for the management of patients with knee osteoarthritis: A randomized double-blind controlled clinical study. International Journal of Rheumatic Diseases. 2012;**15**(2):197-206

[20] Baker KG, Robertson VJ, Duck FAA. A review of therapeutic ultrasound: Biophysical effects. Physical Therapy. 2001;**81**(7):1351-1358

[21] Rutjes AW, Nüesch E, Sterchi R, Jüni P. Therapeutic ultrasound for osteoarthritis of the knee or hip (review). Cochrane Database of Systematic Reviews. 2010;**1**:CD003132

[22] Huang YY, Chen AC, Carroll JD, Hamblin MR. Biphasic dose response in low level light therapy. Dose-Response. 2009;**7**(4):358-383

[23] Hamblin MR, Demidova TN. Mechanisms of low-level light therapy. Proceedings of SPIE. 2006;**6140**: 1-12. Figure 6. Cell signaling pathways induced by LLLT; p. 6

[24] Pallotta RC, Bjordal JM, Frigo L, Leal Junior EC, Teixeira S, Marcos RL, et al. Infrared (810-nm) low-level laser therapy on rat experimental knee inflammation. Lasers in Medical Science. 2012;**27**(1):71-78

[25] Lemos GA, Rissi R, de Souza Pires IL, de Oliveira LP, de Aro AA, Pimentel ER, et al. Low-level laser therapy stimulates tissue repair and reduces the extracellular matrix degradation in rats with induced arthritis in the temporomandibular joint. Lasers in Medical Science. 2016;**31**(6):1051-1059

[26] Barushka O, Yaakobi T, Oron U. Effect of low-energy laser (He-Ne) irradiation on the process of bone repair in the rat tibia. Bone. 1995;**16**(1):47-55

[27] Grassi FR, Ciccolella F, D'Apolito G, Papa F, Iuso A, Salzo AE, et al. Effect of low-level laser irradiation on osteoblast proliferation and bone formation. Journal of Biological Regulators and Homeostatic Agents. 2011;**25**(4):603-614

[28] Saito S, Shimizu N. Stimulatory effects of low-power laser irradiation on bone regeneration in midpalatal suture during expansion in the rat. American Journal of Orthodontics and Dentofacial Orthopedics. 1997;**111**(5):525-532

[29] Almeida-Lopes L, Rigau J, Zângaro RA, Guidugli-Neto J, Jaeger MM. Comparison of the low level laser therapy effects on cultured human gingival fibroblasts proliferation using different irradiance and same fluence. Lasers in Surgery and Medicine. 2001;**29**(2):179-184

[30] Kreisler M, Christoffers AB, Al-Haj H, Willershausen B, d'Hoedt B. Low level 809-nm diode laser-induced in vitro stimulation of the proliferation of human gingival fibroblasts. Lasers in Surgery and Medicine. 2002;**30**(5): 365-369

[31] Medrado AR, Pugliese LS, Reis SR, Andrade ZA. Influence of low level laser therapy on wound healing and its biological action upon myofibroblasts. Lasers in Surgery and Medicine. 2003;**32**(3):239-244

[32] Wang P, Liu C, Yang X, Zhou Y, Wei X, Ji Q, et al. Effects of low level laser therapy on joint pain, synovitis, anabolic

and catabolic factors in a progressive osteoarthritis rabbit model. Lasers in Medical Science. 2014;**29**(6):1875-1885

[33] Brosseau L, Welch V, Wells G, deBie R, Gam A, Harman K, et al. Low level laser therapy for osteoarthritis and rheumatoid arthritis: A metaanalysis, The Journal of Rheumatology. 2000;**27**(8):1961-1969

[34] Al-Rashoud AS, Abboud RJ, Wang W, Wigderowitz C. Efficacy of low-level laser therapy at acupuncture points in knee osteoarthritis: A randomised double blind comparative trial. Physiotherapy. 2014;**100**(3):242-248

[35] Soleimnapour H, Gahramani K, Taheri R, Golzari SE, Safari S, Esfanjani RM, et al. The effect of low-level laser therapy on knee osteoarthritis: Prospective, descriptive study. Lasers in Medical Science. 2014;**29**(5):1695-1700

[36] Baltzer AWA, Stosch D, Seidel F, Ostapczuk MS. Low level laser therapy: A narrative literature review on the efficacy in the treatment of rheumatic orthopaedic conditions. Zeitschrift für Rheumatologie. 2017;**76**(9):806-812

[37] Cashman JN. The mechanisms of action of NSAIDs in analgesia. Drugs. 1996;**52**(5):13-23

[38] Vuilleumier PH, Schliessbach J, Curatolo M. Current evidence for central analgesic effects of NSAIDs: An overview of the literature. Minerva Anestesiologica. 2018;**84**(7):865-870

[39] Haroutiunian S, Drennan DA, Lipman AG. Topical NSAID therapy for musculoskeletal pain. Pain Medicine. 2010;**11**(4):535-549

[40] Anon. Topical Analgesics: A Review of Reviews and a Bit of Perspective. 2005. Available from: www.jr2.ox.ac.uk/Bandolier/Extraforbando/Topextra3.pdf

[41] Sioufi A, Pommier F, Boschet F, Godbillon J, Lavoignat D, Salliere D. Percutaneous absorption of diclofenac in healthy volunteers after single and repeated topical application of diclofenac Emulgel. Biopharmaceutics & Drug Disposition. 1994;**15**(6):441-449

[42] Massey T, Derry S, Moore RA, McQuay HJ. Topical NSAIDs for acute pain in adults. Cochrane Database of Systematic Reviews. 2010;**6**:CD007402

[43] Brunner M, Dehghanyar P, Seigfried B, Martin W, Menke G, Müller M. Favourable dermal penetration of diclofenac after administration to the skin using a novel spray gel formulation. British Journal of Clinical Pharmacology. 2005;**60**(5):573-577

[44] Barthel HR, Haselwood D, Longley S 3rd, Gold MS, Altman RD. Randomized controlled trial of diclofenac sodium gel in knee osteoarthritis. Seminars in Arthritis and Rheumatism. 2009;**39**(3):203-212

[45] Moore RA, Tramer MR, Carroll D, Wiffen PJ, McQuay HJ. Quantitative systematic review of topical applied non-steroidal anti-inflammatory drugs. British Medical Journal. 1998;**316**(7168):333-338

[46] Mason L, Moore RA, Edwards JE, Derry S, McQuay HJ. Topical NSAIDs for chronic musculoskeletal pain: Systematic review and meta-analysis. BMC Musculoskeletal Disorders. 2004;**5**:28

[47] Lin J, Zhang W, Jones A, Doherty M. Efficacy of topical non-steroidal anti-inflammatory drugs in the treatment of osteoarthritis: Meta-analysis of randomised controlled trials. British Medical Journal. 2004;**329**(7461):324

[48] Biswal S, Medhi B, Pandhi P. Long-term efficacy of topical nonsteroidal anti-inflammatory drugs in knee osteoarthritis: Meta-analysis of

randomized placebo controlled clinical trials. The Journal of Rheumatology. 2006;**33**(9):1841-1844

[49] Roth SH, Shainhouse JZ. Efficacy and safety of a topical diclofenac solution (pennsaid) in the treatment of primary osteoarthritis of the knee: A randomized, double-blind, vehicle-controlled clinical trial. Archives of Internal Medicine. 2004;**164**(18):2017-2023

[50] Underwood M, Ashby D, Cross P, Hennessy E, Letley L, Martin J, et al. Advice to use topical or oral ibuprofen for chronic knee pain in older people: Randomised controlled trial and patient preference study. British Medical Journal. 2008;**336**(7636):138-142

[51] Tugwell PS, Wells GA, Shainhouse JZ. Equivalence study of a topical diclofenac solution (pennsaid) compared with oral diclofenac in symptomatic treatment of osteoarthritis of the knee: A randomized controlled trial. The Journal of Rheumatology. 2004;**31**(10):2002-2012

[52] Simon LS, Grierson LM, Naseer Z, Bookman AA, Zev SJ. Efficacy and safety of topical diclofenac containing dimethyl sulfoxide (DMSO) compared with those of topical placebo. DMSO vehicle and oral diclofenac for knee osteoarthritis. Pain. 2009;**143**(3):238-245

[53] Makris UE, Kohler MJ, Fraenkel L. Adverse effects of topical non-steroidal anti-inflammatory drugs in older adults with osteoarthritis: A systematic literature review. The Journal of Rheumatology. 2010;**3**(6):1236-1243

[54] Baron R. Capsaicin and nociception: From basic mechanisms to novel drugs. Lancet. 2000;**356**(9232):785-787

[55] Nolano M, Simone DA, Wendelschafer-Crabb G, Johnson T, Hazen E, Kennedy WR. Topical capsaicin in humans: Parallel loss of epidermal nerve fibres and pain sensation. Pain. 1999;**81**(1-2):135-145

[56] Mason L, Moore RA, Derry S, Edwards JE, McQuay HJ. Systematic review of topical capsaicin for the treatment of chronic pain. British Medical Journal. 2004;**328**(7446):991-994

[57] Zhang W, Moskowitz RW, Nuki G, Abramson S, Altman RD, Arden N, et al. OARSI recommendations for the management of hip and knee osteoarthritis, Part II: OARSI evidence-based, expert consensus guidelines. Osteoarthritis and Cartilage. 2008;**16**(2):137-162

[58] Laslett LL, Jones G. Capsaicin for osteoarthritis pain. Progress in Drug Research. 2014;**68**:277-291

[59] Morton I, Hall J. The Royal Society of Medicine: Medicines. 6th ed. London: Bloomsbury; 2002

[60] Derry S, Matthews PR, Wiffen PJ, Moore RA. Salicylate-containing rubefacients for acute and chronic musculoskeletal pain in adults. Cochrane Database of Systematic Reviews. 2014;**11**:CD007403

[61] The PrescQIPP DROP-List. Bulletin 114. Version 2.1. 2015. Available from: www.prescqipp.info

[62] Burch F, Codding C, Patel N, Sheldon E. Lidocaine 5% patch improves pain, stiffness, and physical function in osteoarthritis pain patients. A prospective, multicenter, open-label effectiveness trial. Osteoarthritis and Cartilage. 2004;**12**(3):253-255

[63] Comer AM, Lamb HM. Lidocaine patch 5%. Drugs. 2000;**59**(2):245-249

[64] Ramamoorthy S, Cidlowski JA. Corticosteroids—Mechanisms of action in health and disease. Rheumatic Diseases Clinics of North America. 2016;**42**(1):15-31

[65] Croxtall JD, Choudhury Q, Flower RJ. Glucocorticoids act within minutes to inhibit recruitment of signalling factors to activated EGF receptors through a receptor-dependent, transcription-independent mechanism. British Journal of Pharmacology. 2000;**130**(2):289-298

[66] Jones A, Doherty M. Intra-articular corticosteroids are effective in osteoarthritis but there are no clinical predictors of response. Annals of the Rheumatic Diseases. 1996;**55**(11):829-832

[67] Gaffney K, Ledingham J, Perry JD. Intra-articular triamcinolone hexacetonide in knee osteoarthritis: Factors influencing the clinical response. Annals of the Rheumatic Diseases. 1995;**54**(5):379-381

[68] Ayral X. Injections in the treatment of osteoarthritis. Best Practice & Research. Clinical Rheumatology. 2001;**15**(4):609-626

[69] Schumacher HR. Aspiration and injection therapies for joints. Arthritis and Rheumatism. 2003;**49**(3):413-420

[70] Pyne D, Ioannou Y, Mootoo R, Bhanji A. Intra-articular steroids in knee osteoarthritis: A comparative study of triamcinolone hexacetonide and methylprednisolone acetate. Clinical Rheumatology. 2004;**23**(2):116-120

[71] Friedman DM, Moore ME. The efficacy of intra-articular steroids in osteoarthritis: A double-blind study. The Journal of Rheumatology. 1980;**7**(6):850-856

[72] Dieppe PA, Sathapatayavongs B, Jones HE, Bacon PA, Ring EF. Intra-articular steroids in osteoarthritis. Rheumatology and Rehabilitation. 1980;**19**(4):212-217

[73] Jüni P, Hari R, Rutjes AW, Fischer R, Silletta MG, Reichenbach S, et al. Intra-articular corticosteroid for knee osteoarthritis. Cochrane Database of Systematic Reviews. 2015;**10**:CD005328

[74] Flanagan J, Casale FF, Thomas TL, Desai KB. Intra-articular injection for pain relief in patients awaiting hip replacement. Annals of The Royal College of Surgeons of England. 1988;**70**(3):156-157

[75] Qvistgaard E, Christensen R, Torp-Pedersen S, Bliddal H. Intra-articular treatment of hip osteoarthritis: A randomized trial of hyaluronic acid, corticosteroid, and isotonic saline. Osteoarthritis and Cartilage. 2006;**14**(2):163-170

[76] Meenagh GK, Patton J, Kynes C, Wright GD. A randomised controlled trial of intra-articular corticosteroid injection of the carpometacarpal joint of the thumb in osteoarthritis. Annals of the Rheumatic Diseases. 2004;**63**(10):1260-1263

[77] Day CS, Gelberman R, Patel AA, Vogt MT, Ditsios K, Boyer MI. Basal joint osteoarthritis of the thumb: A prospective trial of steroid injection and splinting. Journal of Hand Surgery. 2004;**29**(2):247-251

[78] Creamer P. Intra-articular corticosteroid treatment in osteoarthritis. Current Opinion in Rheumatology. 1999;**11**(5):417-421

[79] Kumar N, Newman RJ. Complications of intra- and peri-articular steroid injections. The British Journal of General Practice. 1999;**49**(443):465-466

[80] Habib GS. Systemic effects of intra-articular corticosteroids. Clinical Rheumatology. 2009;**28**(7):749-756

[81] Pattrick M, Doherty M. Facial flushing after intra-articular injection of bupivacaine and methylprednisolone. British Medical Journal. 1987;**295**(6610):1380

[82] Slotkoff A, Clauw D, Nashel D. Effect of soft tissue corticosteroid injection on glucose control in diabetics. Arthritis and Rheumatism. 1994;**37**(9):S347

[83] Papacrhistou G, Anagnostou S, Katsorhis T. The effect of intraarticular hydrocortisone injection on the articular cartilage of rabbits. Acta Orthopaedica Scandinavica. Supplementum. 1997;**275**:132-134

[84] Raynauld JP, Buckland-Wright C, Ward R, Choquette D, Haraoui B, Martel-Pelletier J, et al. Safety and efficacy of long-term intraarticular steroid injections in osteoarthritis of the knee: A randomized, double-blind, placebo-controlled trial. Arthritis and Rheumatism. 2003;**48**(2):370-377

[85] National Institute for Health and Care Excellence. Osteoarthritis: National Clinical Guideline for Care and Management in Adults. London: NICE; 2014. Available from: www.nice.org.uk/CG117

[86] Fife RS. Osteoarthritis: Epidemiology, pathology and pathogenesis. In: Klippel JH, editor. Primer on the Rheumatic Diseases. 11th ed. The Arthritis Foundation: Atlanta; 1997. pp. 216-217

[87] Altman RD, Manjoo A, Fierlinger A, Niazi F, Nicholls M. The mechanism of action for hyaluronic acid treatment in the osteoarthritic knee: A systematic review. BMC Musculoskeletal Disorders. 2015;**16**:321

[88] Mihara M, Hashizume M, Yoshida H, Suzuki M, Shiina M. IL-6/IL-6 receptor system and its role in physiological and pathological conditions. Clinical Science. 2012;**122**(4):143-159

[89] Wobig M, Bach G, Beks P, Dickhut A, Runzheimer J, Schiewger G, et al. The role of elastoviscosity in the efficacy of viscosupplementation for osteoarthritis of the knee: A comparison of hylan G-F 20 and a lower-molecular-weight hyaluronan. Clinical Therapeutics. 1999;**21**(9):1549-1562

[90] Bellamy N, Campbell J, Robinson V, Gee T, Bourne R, Wells G. Viscosupplementation for the treatment of osteoarthritis of the knee. Cochrane Database of Systematic Reviews. 2006;**2**:CD005321

[91] Qvistgaard E, Christensen R, Torp-Pedersen S, Bliddal H. Intra-articular treatment of hip osteoarthritis: A randomized trial of hyaluronic acid, corticosteroid, and isotonic saline. Osteoarthritis and Cartilage. 2006;**14**(2):163-170

[92] Fuchs S, Mönikes R, Wohlmeiner A, Heyse T. Intra-articular hyaluronic acid compared with corticoid injections for the treatment of rhizarthrosis. Osteoarthritis and Cartilage. 2006;**14**(1):82-88

[93] Fox WW, Freed DLJ. Understanding Arthritis. London: Macmillan; 1990

[94] Steindler A, Luck JV. Differential diagnoses of pain in the low back. Journal of the American Medical Association. 1938;**110**:106-113

[95] Travell JG, Simons DG, editors. Myofascial Pain and Dysfunction: The Trigger Point Manual. Baltimore, MD, USA: Williams & Wilkins; 1983. pp. 2-18

[96] Cailliet R. Chronic pain concept. In: Soft Tissue Pain and Disability. Philadelphia, PA, USA: FA Davis; 1977. pp. 25-40

[97] Kim PS. Role of injection therapy: Review of indications for trigger point injections, regional blocks, facet joint injections, and intra-articular injections. Current Opinion in Rheumatology. 2002;**14**(1):52-57

[98] Scott NA, Guo B, Barton PM, Gerwin RD. Trigger point injections for

chronic non-malignant musculoskeletal pain: A systematic review. Pain Medicine. 2009;**10**(1):54-69

[99] Yentür EA, Okcu G, Yegul I. The role of trigger point therapy in knee osteoarthritis. The Pain Clinic. 2003;**15**: 385-390

[100] Sidel N, Abrams MI. Treatment of chronic arthritis: results of vaccine therapy with saline injections used as controls. Journal of the American Medical Association. 1940;**11**:1740-1742

[101] Traut EF, Passarelli EW. Study in the controlled therapy of degenerative arthritis. Archives of Internal Medicine. 1956;**98**(2):181-186

[102] Frost FA, Jessen B, Siggaard-Andersen J. A controlled, double-blind comparison of mepivacaine versus saline injection for myofascial pain. Lancet. 1980;**1**(8167):499-500

[103] Frost FA. Diclofenac versus lidocaine as injection therapy in myofascial pain. Scandinavian Journal of Rheumatology. 1986;**15**:153-156

[104] Byrn C, Olsson I, Falkheden L, Lindh M, Hösterey U, Fogelberg M, et al. Subcutaneous sterile water injections for chronic neck and shoulder pain following whiplash injuries. Lancet. 1993;**341**(8843):449-452

[105] Smith AS, Doré CJ, Dennis L, Julius A, Mackworth-Young CG. A randomised controlled trial of subcutaneous sodium salicylate therapy for osteoarthritis of the thumb. Postgraduate Medical Journal. 2010;**86**(1016):341-345

[106] Kidd BL, Urban LA. Mechanisms of inflammatory pain. British Journal of Anaesthesia. 2001;**87**(1):3-11

[107] Schaible HG, Ebersberger A, Von Banchet GS. Mechanisms of pain in arthritis. Annals of the New York Academy of Sciences. 2002;**966**:343-354

[108] McCarthy GM, McCarty DJ. Effect of topical capsaicin in the therapy of painful osteoarthritis of the hands. The Journal of Rheumatology. 1992;**19**: 604-607

[109] Witt C, Brinkhaus B, Jena S, Linde K, Streng A, Wagenpfeil S, et al. Acupuncture in patients with osteoarthritis of the knee: A randomised trial. Lancet. 2005;**366**(9480):136-143

[110] Molsberger A, Böwing G, Jensen KU, Lorek M. Acupuncture treatment for the relief of gonarthrosis pain—A controlled clinical trial. Der Schmerz. 1994;**8**(1):37-42. (German)

[111] Petrou P, Winkler V, Genti G, Balint G. Double blind trial to evaluate the effect of acupuncture treatment on knee osteoarthritis. The Scandinavian Journal of Acupuncture. 1988;**3**:112-115

[112] Berman BM, Singh BB, Lao L, Langenberg P, Li H, Hadhazy V, et al. A randomized trial of acupuncture as an adjunctive therapy in osteoarthritis of the knee. Rheumatology (Oxford, England). 1999;**38**(4):346-354

[113] Ezzo J, Hadhazy V, Birch S, Kaplan G, Hochberg M, Berman B. Acupuncture for osteoarthritis of the knee: A systematic review. Arthritis and Rheumatism. 2001;**44**(4):819-825

[114] Melchart D, Weidenhammer W, Streng A, Reitmayr S, Hoppe A, Ernst E, et al. Prospective investigation of adverse effects of acupuncture in 97733 patients. Archives of Internal Medicine. 2004;**164**(1):104-105

[115] Berman BM, Lao L, Langenberg P, Lee WL, Gilpin AM, Hochberg MC. Effectiveness of acupuncture as adjunctive therapy in osteoarthritis of the knee. Annals of Internal Medicine. 2004;**141**(12):901-910

[116] Ernst E, White A. Acupuncture: Safety first. British Medical Journal. 1997;**314**(7091):1362

[117] Warden SJ, Hinman RS, Watson MA Jr, Avin KG, Bialocerkowski AE, Crossley KM. Patellar taping and bracing for the treatment of chronic knee pain: A systematic review and meta-analysis. Arthritis and Rheumatism. 2008;**59**(1):73-83

[118] Rannou F, Poiraudeau S, Beaudreuil J. Role of bracing in the management of knee osteoarthritis. Current Opinion in Rheumatology. 2010;**22**(2):218-222

[119] Birmingham TB, Kramer JF, Kirkley A, Inglis JT, Spaulding SJ, Vandervoort AA. Knee bracing for medial compartment osteoarthritis: Effects on proprioception and postural control. Rheumatology (Oxford, England). 2001;**40**(3):285-289

[120] Ramsey DK, Briem K, Axe MJ, Snyder-Mackler L. A mechanical theory for the effectiveness of bracing for medial compartment osteoarthritis of the knee. The Journal of Bone and Joint Surgery. American Volume. 2007;**89**(11):2398-2407

[121] Jordan KM, Arden NK, Doherty M, et al. EULAR Recommendations 2003: An evidence-based approach to the management of knee osteoarthritis: Report of a Task Force of the Standing Committee for International Clinical Studies Including Therapeutic Trials (ESCISIT). Annals of the Rheumatic Diseases. 2003;**62**(12):1145-1155

[122] Altman RD, Hochberg MC, Moskowitz RW, Schnitzer TJ. Recommendations for the medical management of osteoarthritis of the hip and knee: 2000 update. American College of Rheumatology Subcommittee on Osteoarthritis Guidelines. Arthritis & Rheumatology. 2000;**43**(9):1905-1915

[123] Kirkley A, Webster-Bogaert S, Litchfield R, Amendola A, MacDonald S, McCalden R, et al. The effect of bracing on varus gonarthrosis. Journal of Bone and Joint Surgery. 1999;**81**(4):539-548

[124] Brouwer RW, van Raaij TM, Verhaar JA, Coene LN, Bierma-Zeinstra SM. Brace treatment for osteoarthritis of the knee: A prospective randomized multicentre trial. Osteoarthritis and Cartilage. 2006;**14**(8):777-783

[125] Beaudreuil J, Bendaya S, Faucher M, Coudeyre E, Ribinik P, Revel M, et al. Clinical practice guidelines for rest orthosis, knee sleeves, and unloading knee braces in knee osteoarthritis. Joint, Bone, Spine. 2009;**76**(6):629-636

[126] Pollo FE, Otis JC, Backus SI, Warren RF, Wickiewicz TL. Reduction of medial compartment loads with valgus bracing of the osteoarthritic knee. The American Journal of Sports Medicine. 2002;**30**(3):414-421

[127] Giori NJ. Load-shifting brace treatment for osteoarthritis of the knee: A minimum 2 1/2-year follow-up study. Journal of Rehabilitation Research and Development. 2004;**41**(2):187-194

[128] Brouwer RW, Jakma TS, Verhagen AP, Verhaar JA, Bierma-Zeinstra SM. Braces and orthoses for treating osteoarthritis of the knee. Cochrane Database of Systematic Reviews. 2005;**1**:CD004020

[129] Valdes K, Marik T. A systematic review of conservative interventions for osteoarthritis of the hand. Journal of Hand Therapy. 2010;**23**(4):334-350

[130] Bijsterbosch J, Visser W, Kroon HM, Stamm T, Meulenbelt I, Huizinga TW, et al. Thumb base involvement in symptomatic hand osteoarthritis is associated with more pain and functional disability. Annals

of the Rheumatic Diseases. 2010;**69**(3):585-587

[131] Rannou F, Dimet J, Boutron I, Baron G, Fayad F, Macé Y, et al. Splint for base-of-thumb osteoarthritis: A randomized trial. Annals of Internal Medicine. 2009;**150**(10):661-669

[132] Bian L, Hou C, Tous E, Rai R, Mauck RL, Burdick JA. The influence of hyaluronic acid hydrogel crosslinking density and macromolecular diffusivity on human MSC chondrogenesis and hypertrophy. Biomaterials. 2013;**34**(2): 413-421

[133] Huang AH, Farrell MJ, Mauck RL. Mechanics and mechanobiology of mesenchymal stem cell-based engineered cartilage. Journal of Biomechanics. 2010;**43**(1):128-136

[134] Platas J, Guillén MI, del Caz MD, Gomar F, Mirabet V, Alcaraz MJ. Conditioned media from adipose-tissue-derived mesenchymal stem cells downregulate degradative mediators induced by interleukin-1β in osteoarthritic chondrocytes. Mediators of Inflammation. 2013;**2013**:357014

[135] Jukes JM, Both SK, Leusink A, Sterk LM, van Blitterswijk CA, de Boer J. Endochondral bone tissue engineering using embryonic stem cells. Proceedings of the National Academy of Sciences of the United States of America. 2008;**105**(19):6840-6845

[136] Mancuso P, Raman S, Glynn A, Barry F, Murphy JM. Mesenchymal stem cell therapy for osteoarthritis: The critical role of the cell secretome. Frontiers in Bioengineering and Biotechnology. 2019;7:9

[137] Galleu A, Riffo-Vasquez Y, Trento C, Lomas C, Dolcetti L, Cheung TS, et al. Apoptosis in mesenchymal stroma cells induces in vivo recipient-mediated immunomodulation. Science Translational Medicine. 2017;**9**(416):eaam7828

Chapter 8

Simultaneous Bilateral Joint Arthroplasties in Treatment of Osteoarthritis

Aleksandar Radunović, Maja Vulović, Milan Aksić, Ognjen Radunović and Aleksandar Matić

Abstract

Osteoarthrosis is the most common chronic joint condition, the aetiology of which is still not completely clear. Initial phases of disease are treated conservatively applying physical rehabilitation procedures and medications. Advanced stages need surgical treatment with numerous procedures, depending on the joint affected. Joint arthroplasties are procedure of choice, especially for big joints of the extremities. As osteoarthrosis occurs bilaterally very frequently, there are a growing number of patients in need for operation of both joints. Those procedures can be performed under single anaesthesia or staged procedure, with delay between two surgeries. There are many advantages and disadvantages of both approaches cited by different authors. There is consensus of authors in available articles regarding benefits of single-stage procedure: lower cost, shorter hospital stay, single rehabilitation period and better functional results. Authors disagree about safety of a single-stage bilateral procedure as well as incidence of complications and criteria for selection of patients for safe performing of simultaneous procedure.

Keywords: osteoarthrosis, hip, knee, bilateral, simultaneous

1. Introduction

Osteoarthrosis is the most common joint disease in humans [1]. The American College of Rheumatology defines it as a heterogeneous group of joint affections that lead to occurrence of joint symptoms and signs related to damage of joint cartilage integrity, accompanied by changes in subchondral bone and surrounding soft tissues. Aetiology of osteoarthrosis remains only partially known for the time being. It is considered to have multifactorial causes, and its occurrence is a final result of interaction of systemic factors (older age, increased body weight, etc.) as well as local risk factors (mechanical load, injuries, etc.).

Osteoarthrosis can be treated both conservatively and surgically. Conservative treatment options can be divided into pharmacological and non-pharmacological. Those two treatment modalities tend to be combined aiming at achieving best possible results.

Pharmacological therapy includes the use of analgesics, NSAID, corticosteroids, oral drugs based on glucosamine and hyaluronic acid as well as intra-articular injections of sodium hyaluronate and corticosteroids. All the abovementioned therapy modalities have very different results as explained in available reference literature. In the past decade or so, there has been a growing trend of regenerative procedures involving application of platelet-rich plasma (PRP) and stem cell therapy.

Non-pharmacological options include education of patients, reduction of body weight, exercises for muscle strengthening and stretching in order to prevent contractures, application of orthosis as well as different forms of physical rehabilitation.

2. Surgical treatment of osteoarthrosis

2.1 Osteotomies of affected joint(s)

With the development of new materials and new surgical techniques, arthroplasties of joints have become a primary solution in surgical treatment of osteoarthrosis. However, there are still certain indications for osteotomies, especially for osteoarthrosis of lower leg big joints among young adults, aiming to postpone a total joint arthroplasty. Some studies show that at least 40% of patients with performed osteotomies need a total joint arthroplasty only a few years later [2, 3].

2.2 Arthrodesis

Arthrodesis is a surgical fusion of joints. Nowadays it is rarely performed in big joints, mostly as salvage procedure for treating infection after failed arthroplasty. Arthrodesis is more frequently used in treating osteoarthrosis of small joints in the foot.

2.3 Joint arthroplasties

At this moment, joint arthroplasties are the most preferred solution for degenerative changes in big joints, especially the knees, hips and shoulders. There are numerous reports of arthroplasties of these three joints in last few decades, showing excellent functional results and patient satisfaction. As about elbows, ankles, and small joints of the hands and feet, reported arthroplasty outcomes are still not comparable with those in the hips, knees and shoulders.

There are many different forms of joint arthroplasties regarding types of fixation, articular surfaces and materials used for fabricating artificial joints, regardless of whether only one or both articular surfaces of the joint are involved in arthroplasty.

3. Simultaneous bilateral joint arthroplasties

When discussing bilateral joint arthroplasties performed as a single procedure, we are exclusively considering hip and knee arthroplasties. A single-stage bilateral arthroplasties of other joints are not routinely performed, and there are only a few articles dealing with patients when both shoulders were operated in a single procedure. In addition to this, a number of patients mentioned in those articles are quite small [4, 5].

3.1 A single-stage bilateral hip and knee arthroplasty

Osteoarthrosis of the hip (coxarthrosis) occurs at 4% of the population, and 40–70% percent of patients with coxarthrosis have both hips affected [6, 7] (**Figure 1**). It is considered that 97% of patients with bilateral coxarthrosis will be in need for arthroplasty of the second hip as well [8] (**Figure 2**). With osteoarthrosis

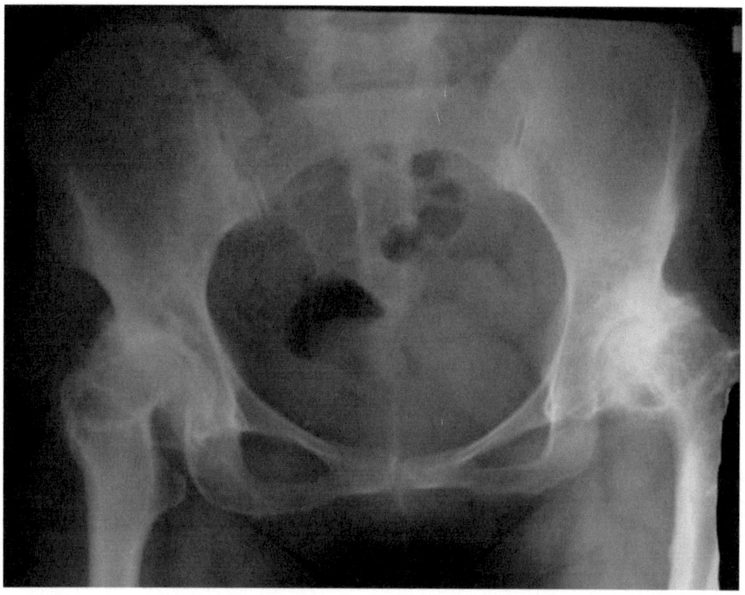

Figure 1.
Bilateral coxarthrosis.

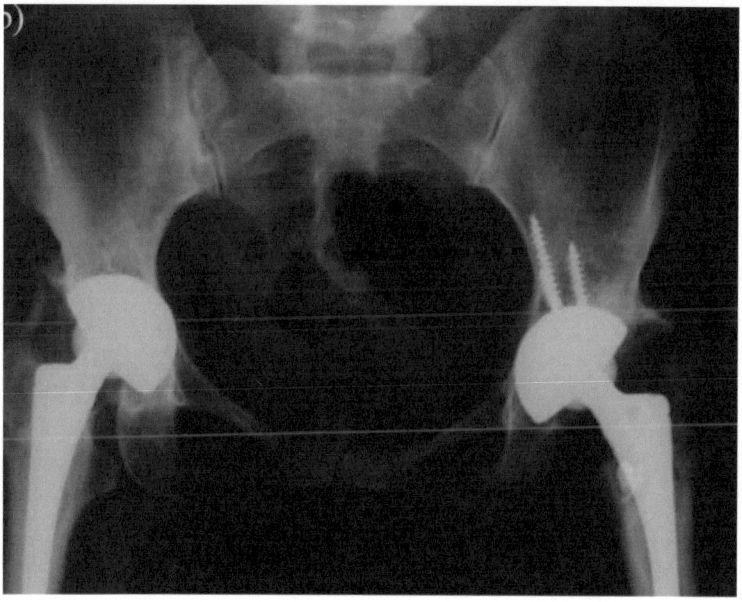

Figure 2.
Simultaneous bilateral total hip arthroplasty.

of the knee (gonarthrosis), it is estimated that 10% of patients older than 55 years have clinical symptoms of gonarthrosis [9], with 30–50% of patients having both knees affected and will be in need of bilateral surgery [10, 11] (**Figures 3** and **4**). Patients with bilateral hip or knee osteoarthritis can be surgically treated in a single procedure, by replacing both hip and knee joints under single anaesthesia, or they could be treated in a two-stage procedure with a break between two procedures. Period between two procedures significantly differs among authors. Having in mind differences among authors when it comes to bilateral hip and knee arthroplasties in a single procedure, we shall analyse them separately.

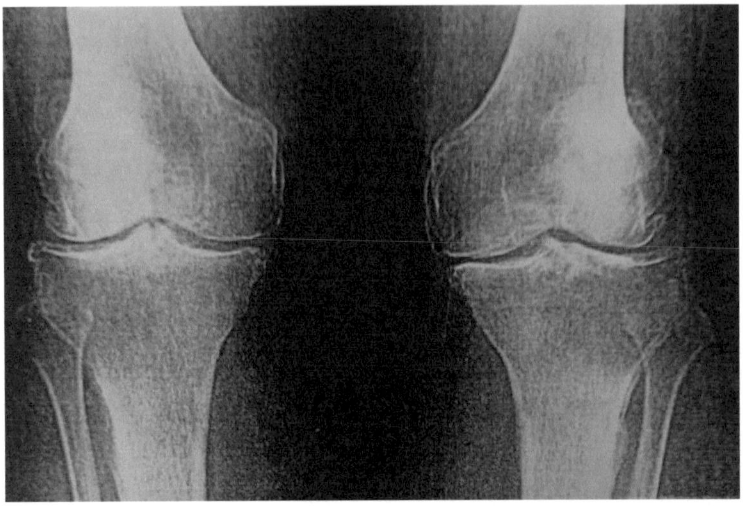

Figure 3.
Bilateral gonarthrosis.

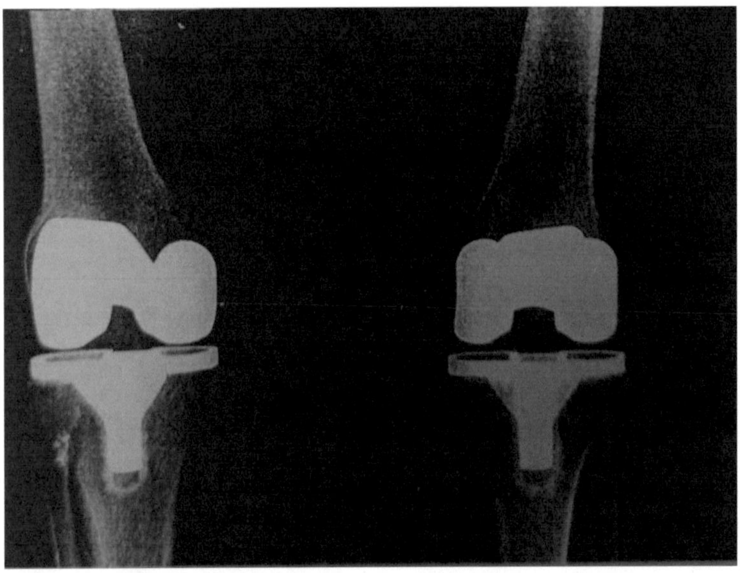

Figure 4.
Simultaneous bilateral knee arthroplasty.

3.2 Simultaneous bilateral total hip arthroplasty

The first simultaneous bilateral total hip arthroplasty was published in 1967 [12]. Jaffe and Charnley published an article in 1971, analysing results of this procedure in 50 patients [13]. Authors found minimally increased risk of complications in a simultaneous group compared to a staged group and noticed advantages of the simultaneous procedure: a single anaesthesia, a single rehabilitation period and shorter hospital days (unlike two hospital slots in a staged procedure). In the succeeding years, multiple authors will have published their results with performing a single-stage bilateral total hip arthroplasty, with lack of consensus regarding safety of procedure, patient selection and frequency of complications. At the same time, authors agreed about benefits of this simultaneous procedure: a significantly better functional recovery and rehabilitation. Some authors have even claimed that a full functional recovery of patient is possible only after implantation of endo-prosthesis in both hips and that functional scores on operated hips are lower if only one hip is operated than in patients with both hips operated in the same procedure [14]. Patients operated in a single procedure achieved better range of movement and better functional satisfaction without significant difference in pain [15]. There are also discrepancies when it comes to the period of time recommended between two surgeries in a staged procedure. Most authors prefer a period ranging from 3 to 6 months between two hip replacements. There was also a strategy of staged surgery during same hospitalization within 7–10 days between two operations. This one has however been abandoned due to significantly increased number of complications reported in majority of studies.

Authors unanimously agree that simultaneous procedure decreases hospital expenses, numbers of hospital days as well as length of rehabilitation [16–22]. It is estimated that hospital costs are reduced by 24–35%. Some authors quote shorter sick leave from work as an additional advantage. There are no studies that have analysed additional expenses (home care services, public services for patient care); hence we may assume that that real savings are even higher.

While discussing financial side effects of the procedure itself, it is interesting to mention that some authors fail to recommend performing a single-stage procedure due to lower income for the surgeon and hospital [23, 24].

Authors' opinions differ regarding selection of patients as well as the type and frequency of complications. Comorbidity is the most important factor when deciding about a safe performance of a bilateral single-stage procedure. Some authors use general determinants such as patients without significant comorbidity, with good general health and who are younger and healthier [17, 25–27].

While analysing articles that tried to objectivize selection of patients, it is noticeable that American Society of Anesthesiologists (ASA) scoring system is almost exclusively used (see below).

- **ASA 1**: A normal healthy patient.
- **ASA 2**: A patient with a mild systemic disease.
- **ASA 3**: A patient with a severe systemic disease that is not life-threatening.
- **ASA 4**: A patient with a severe systemic disease that is a constant threat to life.
- **ASA 5**: A moribund patient who is not expected to survive without the operation.
- **ASA 6**: A declared brain-dead patient whose organs are being removed for donor purposes.

Authors' opinions about groups of ASA scoring systems eligible for safe performance of bilateral single-stage surgery differ as well. Some recommend performing a simultaneous procedure with ASA 1 and 2 [28–30], others suggest this surgery on patients from ASA 1–4 groups [31], some of them say those are patients in ASA 1 and 2 and probably ASA 3 and 4, while certain authors find no differences in complications with patients belonging to ASA 1–3 [32].

One of the major issues with bilateral simultaneous procedure was a theoretical possibility of a higher incidence of thromboembolic complications caused by a prolonged surgical procedure as one of the best-known triggers for this kind of complication [27, 33]. Earlier publications dealing with simultaneous bilateral hip arthroplasty reported a higher rate of pulmonary embolism and a slightly higher mortality rate while performing this procedure [33–35]. Improvements in surgical technique, anaesthesiology (introduction of hypotensive anaesthesia), anticoagulant therapy and early mobilisation showed decrease in numbers of reported complications of this type. Berend and Glait [36, 37] found increased incidence rate of pulmonary thromboembolism, while majority of other authors did not mention similar findings [20, 38–41]. Some of the authors who failed to find any thromboembolic complications in their series of simultaneous procedures explain this as a better adaptation of a patient to mobilisation protocols when both hips are operated.

Majority of authors reported higher need for transfusion in a simultaneous group [20, 24, 29, 32, 38, 42, 43]. Bhan found lower estimated blood loss in simultaneous group but higher number of transfusions [19]. He explained that in a staged group, blood loss is a sum of losses in two surgeries that are separated long enough for organism to compensate loss from first surgery. Some authors did not discover any increased blood loss in a simultaneous group [17, 25, 37, 44]. Glait pointed out that an increased need for transfusion can be expected if a simultaneous procedure is performed by a less experienced surgeon [37].

3.3 Simultaneous bilateral total knee replacement

While history of bilateral total hip replacement is very well documented, there are almost no papers of a single-stage total knee replacement background. There is a trend of growing number of performed TKA. In the period from 1990 to 2004, number of bilateral total knee replacements doubled and even tripled in female population [45].

Similar to bilateral simultaneous hip arthroplasties, there are certain differences among authors regarding safety of the procedure, potential complications and consensus over its benefits. Overall savings from simultaneous procedure are estimated to be 20–58% with the following contributing factors: fewer hospital days, single medical consultations, single anaesthesia and single rehabilitation period [18, 46]. It is also found by majority of authors that patients in a single-stage group experience equal or better functional result and satisfaction [47, 48]. In one study, 95% of patients would rather choose a single-stage procedure all over again, demonstrating high level of satisfaction [46]. Differences among authors apply to potential increased risk of systemic and local complications, as well as to mortality rate following the procedure itself. Some register studies (the USA and Sweden) found increased morbidity and mortality rate [49, 50], while data from New Zealand arthroplasty registry show no differences between two procedures in same terms [51]. Many authors have discovered with their series of patients an increased risk in systemic complications in a single-stage group [52–55], while a few found no difference in the incidence of complications [47, 56–58]. As per selection of patients, there are only several articles recommending application of the scoring system (ASA, see above). Hadley et al. recommend performing the procedure only in ASA 1 and 2 groups [58], while several authors say this procedure is safe with ASA 1–3 groups as well [59–61]. All authors agree there is an increased blood loss in a simultaneous group [52, 58, 62].

4. Conclusion

While planning and selecting patients with bilateral osteoarthritis of big joints, it is essential to balance between medical and economic efficiency of simultaneous bilateral procedures and safety of patients. As majority of patients in need of bilateral surgery have significant comorbidity, it is of crucial importance to standardise perioperative protocols for selection and follow-up of patients. Multidisciplinary approach in a patient perception is of upmost importance; hence it is recommended this procedure is performed in facilities enabling this and by highly trained and experienced surgeons.

Author details

Aleksandar Radunović[1]*, Maja Vulović[2], Milan Aksić[3], Ognjen Radunović[4] and Aleksandar Matić[5]

1 Clinic for Orthopedic Surgery and Traumatology, Military Medical Academy, Belgrade, Serbia

2 Department of Anatomy, Faculty of Medical Sciences, University of Kragujevac, Serbia

3 Institute of Anatomy "Niko Miljanić", Serbia

4 Medical Faculty, University of Belgrade, Serbia

5 Department of Surgery, Faculty of medical sciences, Clinic for Orthopedic Surgery and Traumatology, Kragujevac, Serbia

*Address all correspondence to: aradunovic@yahoo.com

References

[1] Hochberg MC, Silman AJ, Smolen JS, Weinblatt ME, Weisman MH, editors. Rheumatology. 3rd ed. London: Elsevier Limited; 2003

[2] Schramm M, Hohmann D, Radespiel-Troger M, Pitto RP. Treatment of the dysplastic acetabulum with Wagner spherical osteotomy: A study of patients followed for a minimum of twenty years. The Journal of Bone and Joint Surgery. American Volume. 2003;**85A**:808-814

[3] Steppacher SD, Tannast M, Ganz R, Siebenrock KA. Mean 20-year follow-up of Bernese peri-acetabular osteotomy. Clinical Orthopaedics and Related Research. 2008;**466**:1633-1644

[4] Gerber C, Lingenfelter EJ, Reischl N, Sukthankar A. Single-stage bilateral total shoulder arthroplasty. Journal of Bone and Joint Surgery (British). 2006;**88-B**:751-755

[5] Feroussis JC, Papaspiliopoulos A, Kitsios E, Asprogenidis T, Kiriakos A, Tzoras N. Single stage bilateral total shoulder arthroplasty. Orthopaedic Proceedings; Published Online: 21 February 2018;**92-B**(Suppl IV):574

[6] Allen K, Golightly Y. Epidemiology of osteoarthritis: State of the evidence. Current Opinion in Rheumatology. 2015;**27**(3):276-283

[7] Chitnavis J, Sinsheimer JS, Suchard MA, Clipsham K, Carr AJ. End-stage coxarthrosis and gonarthrosis: Aetiology, clinical patterns and radiological features of idiopathic osteoarthritis. Rheumatology. 2000;**39**:612-619

[8] Sayeed SA, Johnson AJ, Jaffe DE, Mont MA. Incidence of contralateral THA after index THA for osteoarthritis. Clinical Orthopaedics and Related Research. 2012;**470**(2):535-540

[9] Peat G, McCarney R, Croft P. Knee pain and osteoarthritis in older adults: A review of community burden and current use of health care. Annals of the Rheumatic Diseases. 2001;**60**:91-97

[10] Liu TK, Chen SH. Simultaneous bilateral total knee arthroplasty in a single procedure. International Orthopaedics. 1998;**22**(6):390-393

[11] Hussain N, Chien T, Hussain F, Bookwala A, Simunovic N, Shetty V, et al. Simultaneous vs staged bilateral total knee arthroplasty. HSS Journal. 2013;**9**(1):50-59

[12] Lazansky M. A Study of Bilateral Low Friction Arthroplasty. Internal Publication No. 3. Centre for Hip Surgery, Wrightington Hospital: Appley Bridge, UK; 1967

[13] Jaffe WL, Charnley J. Bilateral Charnley low-friction arthroplasty as a single operative procedure: A report of fifty cases. Bulletin of the Hospital for Joint Diseases. 1971;**32**:198

[14] Wykman A, Olsson E. Walking ability after total hip arthroplasty: A comparison of gait analysis in unilateral and bilateral cases. Journal of Bone and Joint Surgery. British Volume (London). 1992;**74**:53

[15] Yoshii T, Jinno T, Morita S, Koga D, Matsubara M, Okawa A, et al. Postoperative hip motion and functional recovery after simultaneous bilateral total hip arthroplasty for bilateral osteoarthritis. Journal of Orthopaedic Science. 2009;**14**:161-166

[16] Alfaro-Adrián J, Bayona F, Rech JA, Murray W. One- or two-stage bilateral total hip replacement. The Journal of Arthroplasty. 1999;**14**:439-445

[17] Parvizi J, Tarity TD, Ednan Sheikh E, Sharkey PF, Hozack WJ,

Rothman RH. Bilateral total hip arthroplasty. One-stage versus two-stage procedures. Clinical Orthopaedics and Related Research. 2006;**453**:137-141

[18] Reuben JD, Meyers SJ, Cox DD, et al. Cost comparison between bilateral simultaneous, staged, and unilateral total joint arthroplasty. The Journal of Arthroplasty. 1998;**13**:172

[19] Bhan S, Pankaj A, Malhotra R. One- or two-stage bilateral total hip arthroplasty: A prospective, randomised, controlled study in an Asian population. Journal of Bone and Joint Surgery. British Volume (London). 2006;**88-B**:298-303

[20] Tsiridis E, Pavlou G, Charity J, Tsiridis E, Gie G, West R. The safety and efficacy of bilateral simultaneous total hip replacement an analysis of 2063 cases. Journal of Bone and Joint Surgery. British Volume (London). 2008;**90-B**:1005-1012

[21] Seol JH, Park KS, Yoon TR. Postoperative complications and cost-effectiveness of simultaneous and staged bilateral total hip arthroplasty using a modified minimally invasive two- incision technique. Hip & Pelvis. 2015;**27**(2):77-82

[22] Rolfson O, Digas G, Herberts P, Karrholm J, Borgstrom F, et al. One-stage bilateral total hip replacement is cost-saving. Journal of Orthopedics and Muscular System. 2014;**3**:175

[23] Trojani C, Chaumet-Lagrange V-A, Hovorka E, Carles M, Boileau P. Simultaneous bilateral total hip arthroplasty: Literature review and preliminary results. Revue de Chirurgie Orthopédique et Réparatrice de l'Appareil Moteur. 2006;**92**(8):760-767

[24] Berend KR, Lombardi AV Jr, Adams JB. Simultaneous vs staged cementless bilateral total hip arthroplasty: Perioperative risk comparison. The Journal of Arthroplasty. 2007;**22**(6):111-115

[25] Aghayev E, Beck A, Staub L, Dietrich D, Melloh M, Orljanski W, et al. Simultaneous bilateral hip replacement reveals superior outcome and fewer complications than two-stage procedures: A prospective study including 1819 patients and 5801 follow-ups from a total joint replacement registry. BMC Musculoskeletal Disorders. 2010;**11**:245-255

[26] Popović Z, Rajović J, Radunović A. Total bilateral hip arthroplasty in one surgical procedure. Vojnosanitetski Pregled (Military Medical Review in English). 2007;**64**(10):697-700

[27] Macaulay W, Salvati EA, Sculco TP, Pellicci PM. Single-stage bilateral total hip arthroplasty. The Journal of the American Academy of Orthopaedic Surgeons. 2002;**10**(3):217-221

[28] Trojani C, Ollone T, Saragaglia D, Vielpeau C, Carles M, Prudhon L. One stage bilateral total hip arthroplasty: Functional outcome and complications in 112 patients. Orthopaedics & Traumatology, Surgery & Research. 2012;**98**(6):120-123

[29] Lamo-Espinosa J, Troncoso S, Valentí-Azcarate A, Dıaz de Rada P, Valentı JR. Clinical and radiological short-term complications after single stage bilateral uncemented total hip arthroplasty. Musculoskeletal Surgery. 2015;**99**(1):67-73

[30] Romagnoli S, Zacchetti S, Perazzo P, Verde F, Banfi G, Vigano M. Simultaneous bilateral total hip arthroplasties do not lead to higher complication or allogeneic transfusion rates compared to unilateral procedures. International Orthopaedics. 2013;**37**(11):2125-2130

[31] Garland A, Rolfson O, Garellick G, Kärrholm J, Hailer N. Early postoperative

mortality after simultaneous or staged bilateral primary total hip arthroplasty: An observational register study from the Swedish hip arthroplasty register. BMC Musculoskeletal Disorders. 2015;**16**(1):263-272

[32] Radunovic A. Clinical safety of single stage bilateral cementless hip arthroplasty [PhD thesis]. Serbia: Medical Faculty, University of Kragujevac; 2018

[33] Ritter MA, Campbell ED. Direct comparison between bilaterally implanted cemented and uncemented total hip replacements in six patients. Clinical Orthopaedics. 1986;**207**:77-82

[34] Ritter MA, Stringer EA. Bilateral total hip arthroplasty: A single procedure. Clinical Orthopaedics. 1980;**149**:185

[35] Ritter MA, Randolph JC. Bilateral total hip arthroplasty: A simultaneous procedure. Acta Odontologica Scandinavica. 1976;**47**(2):203-208

[36] Berend ME, Ritter MA, Harty LD, et al. Simultaneous bilateral versus unilateral total hip arthroplasty an outcome analysis. The Journal of Arthroplasty. 2005;**20**:421-426

[37] Glait S, Khatib O, Bansal A, Hochfelder J, Slover J. Comparing the incidence and clinical data for simultaneous bilateral versus unilateral total hip arthroplasty in New York state between 1990 and 2010. The Journal of Arthroplasty. 2015;**30**(11):1887-1891

[38] Kim YH, Kwon OR, Kim JS. Is one-stage bilateral sequential total hip replacement as safe as unilateral total hip replacement? Journal of Bone and Joint Surgery (British). 2009;**91-B**:316-320

[39] Eggli S, Huckell CB, Ganz R. Bilateral total hip arthroplasty: One stage versus two-stage procedure. Clinical Orthopaedics. 1996;**328**:108-118

[40] Lorenze M, Huo MH, Zatorski LE, Keggi KJ. A comparison of the cost effectiveness of one- stage versus two-stage bilateral total hip replacement. Orthopaedics. 1998;**21**:1249-1252

[41] Cammisa FPOBS Jr, Salvati EA, Sculco TP, Wilson PD Jr, Ranawat CS, Pellicci PM, et al. One-stage bilateral total hip arthroplasty. A prospective study of perioperative morbidity. The Orthopedic Clinics of North America. 1988;**19**(3):657-668

[42] Parvizi J, Pour AE, Peak L, Sharkey P, Hozack W, Rothman R. One-stage bilateral total hip arthroplasty compared with unilateral total hip arthroplasty. The Journal of Arthroplasty. 2006;**21**(6 Suppl 2):26-31

[43] Schäfer M, Elke R, Young JR, Gancs P, Kindler CH. Safety of one-stage bilateral hip and knee arthroplasties under regional anaesthesia and routine anaesthetic monitoring. Journal of Bone and Joint Surgery (British). 2005;**87-B**:1134-1139

[44] Diwanji SR, Park KS, Yoon TR, Seo HY, Wie JS. Bilateral simultaneous two-incision mini mal invasive total hip arthroplasty. Journal of Orthopaedic Science. 2009;**14**:517-524

[45] Memtsoudis SG, Besculides MC, Reid S, Gaber-Baylis LK, González Della Valle A. Trends in bilateral total knee arthroplasties: 153,259 discharges between 1990 and 2004. Clinical Orthopaedics and Related Research. 2009;**467**(6):1568-1576

[46] Leonard L, Williamson DM, Ivory JP, Jennison C. An evaluation of the safety and efficacy of simultaneous bilateral total knee arthroplasty. The Journal of Arthroplasty. 2003;**18**(8):972-978

[47] Kim YH, Choi YW, Kim JS. Simultaneous bilateral sequential total knee replacement is as safe as unilateral total knee replacement. Journal of

Bone and Joint Surgery. British Volume (London). 2009;**91**(1):64-68

[48] March LM, Cross M, Tribe KL, et al. Two knees or not two knees? Patient costs and outcomes following bilateral and unilateral total knee joint replacement surgery for OA. Osteoarthritis and Cartilage. 2004;**12**(5):400-408

[49] Bolognesi MP, Watters TS, Attarian DE, Wellman SS, Setoguchi S. Simultaneous vs staged bilateral total knee arthroplasty among medicare beneficiaries, 2000-2009. The Journal of Arthroplasty. 2013;**28**:87-91

[50] Stefansdottir A, Lidgren L, Robertsson O. Higher early mortality with simultaneous rather than staged bilateral TKAs: Results from the Swedish knee arthroplasty register. Clinical Orthopaedics and Related Research. 2008;**466**:3066-3070

[51] Hooper GJ, Hooper NM, Rothwell AG, Hobbs T. Bilateral total joint arthroplasty: The early results from the New Zealand National Joint Registry. The Journal of Arthroplasty. 2009;**24**:1174-1177

[52] Memtsoudis SG, Ma Y, González Della Valle A, et al. Perioperative outcomes after unilateral and bilateral total knee arthroplasty. Anesthesiology. 2009;**111**(6):1206-1216

[53] Ritter MA, Harty LD, Davis KE, Meding JB, Berend M. Simultaneous bilateral, staged bilateral, and unilateral total knee arthroplasty. A survival analysis. The Journal of Bone and Joint Surgery. American Volume. 2003;**85-A**(8):1532-1537

[54] Hutchinson JR, Parish EN, Cross MJ. A comparison of bilateral uncemented total knee arthroplasty: Simultaneous or staged? Journal of Bone and Joint Surgery. British Volume (London). 2006;**88**(1):40-43

[55] Luscombe JC, Theivendran K, Abudu A, Carter SR. The relative safety of one-stage bilateral total knee arthroplasty. International Orthopaedics. 2009;**33**(1):101-104

[56] Bini SA, Khatod M, Inacio MC, Paxton EW. Same-day versus staged bilateral total knee arthroplasty poses no increase in complications in 6,672 primary procedures. The Journal of Arthroplasty. 2014;**29**(4):694-697

[57] Shin YH, Kim MH, Ko JS, Park JA. The safety of simultaneous bilateral versus unilateral total knee arthroplasty: The experience in a Korean hospital. Singapore Medical Journal. 2010;**51**:44-49

[58] Hadley S, Day M, Schwarzkopf R, Smith A, Slover J, Zuckerman J. Is simultaneous bilateral total knee arthroplasty (BTKA) as safe as staged BTKA? American Journal of Orthopedics (Belle Mead, N.J.). 2017;**46**(4):E224-E229

[59] Memtsoudis SG, Ma Y, Chiu YL, Poultsides L, Gonzalez Della Valle A, Mazumdar M. Bilateral total knee arthroplasty: Risk factors for major morbidity and mortality. Anesthesia and Analgesia. 2011;**113**(4):784-790

[60] Noble J, Goodall JR, Noble DJ. Simultaneous bilateral total knee replacement: A persistent controversy. The Knee. 2009;**16**(6):420-426

[61] Yoon HS, Han CD, Yang IH. Comparison of simultaneous bilateral and staged bilateral total knee arthroplasty in terms of perioperative complications. The Journal of Arthroplasty. 2010;**25**(2):179-185

[62] Breakwell LM, Getty CJ, Dobson P. The efficacy of autologous blood transfusion in bilateral total knee arthroplasty. The Knee. 2000;**7**(3):145-147